Be Well... STAY WELL!

JOAN A. FRIEDRICH, Ph.D.

Keats Publishing, Inc. New Canaan, Connecticut

Be Well ... Stay Well! is not intended as medical advice. Its intention is solely informational and educational. Please consult a medical or health professional should the need for one be indicated.

BE WELL ... STAY WELL!

Copyright © 1989 by Joan A. Friedrich
All Rights Reserved. No part of this book may be copied or reproduced in any form without the written permission of the publisher.

Library of Congress Cataloging-in-Publication Data

Friedrich, Joan A.
   Be well ... stay well.

   Includes bibliographical references and index.
   1. Health. 2. Nutrition. 3. Exercise.
I. Title.
RA776.F857   1989   613   88-8946
ISBN 0-87983-478-1

Printed in the United States of America
Keats/Pivot Health Books are published by
Keats Publishing, Inc.
27 Pine Street (PO Box 876)
New Canaan, Connecticut 06840

Be Well... STAY WELL!

Other Keats Books of Related Interest

The Additives Book, Beatrice Trum Hunter
Diet and Disease (Updated), E. Cheraskin, M.D., D.M.D., W. M. Ringsdorf, Jr., D.M.D. and J. W. Clark, D.D.S.
The Do-It-Yourself Allergy Analysis Handbook, Kate Ludeman, Ph.D. and Louise Henderson with Henry S. Basayne
Environmental Medicine, Natalie Golos, James F. O'Shea, M.D. and Francis J. Waickman, M.D. with Frances Golos Golbitz
Everywoman's Every Day Exercise and Nutrition Plan, Barbara Hegne
The Calcium Plus Workbook, Evelyn P. Whitlock, M.D.
Home Study Course in the New Nutrition, Ruth Yale Long, Ph.D.
How to Improve Your Health, Linda Clark
Know Your Nutrition, Linda Clark
The Nutrition Desk Reference, Robert H. Garrison, Jr., M.A., R.Ph. and Elizabeth Somer, M.A., R.D.
Nutrition and Your Immune System, Carlson Wade
Orthomolecular Nutrition, Abram Hoffer, M.D., Ph.D. and Morton Walker, D.P.M.
Vitamins, Minerals and Other Supplements, Carlson Wade
Your Family Tree Connection, Chris S. Reading, M.D. and Ross S. Meillon

The Self-Care Health Library

Assess Your Own Nutritional Status, Jeffrey Bland, Ph.D.
Evaluate Your Own Biochemical Individuality, **Jeffrey Bland, Ph.D.**
Intestinal Toxicity and Inner Cleansing, Jeffrey Bland, Ph.D.
Recognize and Manage Your Allergies, Doris J. Rapp, M.D.

In Memory of

DR. ELLEN M. KRYLOWSKI
(1952–1984)

For the many blessings of the friendship we
shared and the many lives she so profoundly touched.

CONTENTS

Understanding Wellness 1
Part One: **Nutrition as a Basis of Good Health** 5
   THE RISKS OF OUR DECLINING DIET 7
      Senate Select Committee Recommendations, 9
   FOOD FACTORS ENDANGERING YOUR WELLNESS 11
      Sugars, 11 • Fats and Cholesterol, 13 • Sodium (Salt), 18 • Food Additives, 21 • Toxic Metals, 22 • Overprocessed and Overcooked Foods, 24 • Insecticide-Treated or Irradiated Foods, 25 • Caffeine, 27 • Tap Water, 29 • Alcohol, 30 • Sensitivities and Allergies, 34 • Special Alert for Asthmatics and the Sulfite-Sensitive, 41
   ESSENTIALS OF BASIC HEALTHY EATING 43
      "The Undesirables," 43 • "The Desirables," 44 • Structuring Your Diet, 48 • Bulking Up with Fiber for Better Health, 50 • Vitamins and Minerals, 50 • Amino Acids, 54 • Supplements and Drugs: Some Don't Mix, 57 • Tyramine-Rich Foods—Dietary Restriction for Migraine and MAO Patients, 59

Part Two: **Balancing Your Lifestyle with Exercise and Living** 61
   WELLNESS THROUGH MORE BALANCED LIVING 63
      How to Find Your Training Heart Rate, 64 • Your Resting Heart Rate, 65 • How to Take Your Exercise Pulse Rate, 66 • Exercise—Some Varied Forms, 66 • How to Measure Your Body, 70 •

GETTING IN TOUCH WITH THE INNER SELF 73
    Life Stressors, 74 • Social Readjustment Scale, 74 •
    10 Warning Signs of Mental Illness, 77 • Common
    Stress Indicators and Potential Linked Conditions, 78
    • Characteristic Behaviors, 81 • Help Yourself Ways
    to De-Stress, 82 • Professional Assistance to Help
    De-Stress, 83 • Directions for the Complete Breath,
    84 • Breathing Phrases, 85
GLOSSARY OF COMMON HEALTH TERMS 87
IMPORTANT RESOURCES 97
    Organic Food by Mail, 97 • Learning and Trans-
    formational Programs, 98 • Helpful Hotlines, 99 •
    Sources of Important Health-Related Information, 100
    • Rejuvenating Getaways and Escapes, 104
REFERENCES 112
INDEX 115

UNDERSTANDING WELLNESS

"In order to cure the human body it is necessary to know the whole of things."
—HIPPOCRATES

ACHIEVING AND MAINTAINING good health are often concepts that seem elusively out of reach to many people. The term, "health," has so many connotations that most people are not completely sure of what it actually means. Looking at the work of the Constitution of the World Health Organization, we find that health is more than just the absence of disease or infirmity—it is vastly dependent upon our entire way of living.

Most people are aware that becoming ill can be predicted by typically obvious errors in our styles of living. Smoking, for example, is a major risk for heart and lung diseases and various forms of cancer. Alcohol is a factor in nearly half of all traffic fatalities, half of all homicides and a major cause in health conditions affecting the liver, immunity, nervous system, gastrointestinal tract and many other internal functions. Yet few people equate health with a total assessment of their diet, living habits, psychological attitudes and levels of emotional balance. Most individuals fail to see that health is interdependent on many factors.

Diet, for example, accounts for at least six of the major causes of disease today (heart disease, some cancers, stroke and hypertension, diabetes, arteriosclerosis and cirrhosis of the liver), while stress, especially when chronic, may lead to many forms of deterioration.

We now know that inappropriate physical and emotional responses to stress cannot only lead to feelings of anxiety, hostility and depression, but also to virtually every medical condition, ranging from colds to cancer.

This conceptual and all-encompassing view of health is what is now more commonly known as holistic medicine. A holistic view of health takes into account every possible factor that contributes to an individual's level of health and well-being, both physically and emotionally, and recognizes the reciprocal interaction of body, mind and spirit in the achievement and maintenance of optimum levels of health and wellness.

In this view, body symptoms (referred to medically and psychologically as psychic pain) are more than just black and white diagnoses; they are messages we give ourselves to change our diet, reduce stress, exercise, be more self-aware, express our deep needs and emotions, change our work or living arrangements, increase our levels of maturity and responsibility or address the often neglected nourishment we need from the emotional and spiritual dimensions of our lives. Wellness is dependent upon positive and

Understanding Wellness

assertive steps that enhance our levels of health on many levels.

Wellness requires confidence in the future and active participation in creating a healthier body and mind. Those who aspire to have high levels of wellness make constructive decisions about their lives and their health, and take active steps to improve and maintain them through healthier habits, greater self-esteem and more balanced ways of living.

Well people are fit people, in both body and mind. They are aware of the importance of knowing what total health is all about. They know the steps and factors involved in good health, and they practice these with responsible and active participation. They realize we don't catch a migraine headache or coronary heart disease, but that our lifestyles have a great deal to do with what we manifest as bodily ills. They recognize the importance of sensible balance, too. They clearly see the relationship between all the dimensions of life and of themselves, and place equal importance on every factor. They see and live life with optimism, hope and faith, and discard the negativity, obsessiveness and destructive habits, patterns and dependencies that can foster a halt in their mature growth and lead to the deterioration of the quality of their life or of their physical and mental health. They are able to see themselves more realistically and regularly ask themselves, "How healthy am I?" by assessing how active they are in self-improvement, how good their diet is, how appropriate their level of exercise is, how peaceful and content they feel (physically, emotionally, spiritually), how effectively and responsibly they care for themselves (and others), and how actively they work along with their medical and health-care provider in achieving the best possible level of wellness.

Part One: NUTRITION AS A BASIS OF GOOD HEALTH

Let your food be your medicine and your medicine be your food.
—HIPPOCRATES

THE RISKS OF OUR DECLINING DIET

DURING the last eighty years the American diet has been radically declining. Today's menu may, at times, resemble a traditional fare in its description, yet in reality it bears little nutritional resemblance to the quality that our grandparents enjoyed. Unlike our ancestors, whose diet consisted primarily of locally grown and pesticide-free whole-grain products, fruits, vegetables, legumes, fish, game, etc., many of us consume about ninety-five percent of our diet from foods that are treated, sprayed or processed in some way. Our grains are milled, flaked, puffed or extracted; vegetables are heated and salted; fruits are sliced, diced, packed and syruped; oils are altered; livestock products (poultry, dairy, meats) are filled with residues of antibiotics, hormones and other potentially risky agents. We must even wonder about the quality of much of our seafood and the water we drink, because of the vastness of industrial and water pollution. To make matters worse, most of our commercial food products supply us with many hidden salts, sugars and fats, and a broad array of dyes, coloring agents, flavor enhancers and preservatives, all of which may compromise our health. These can create serious risks for both the lifestyle- and diet-related "degenerative diseases" (obesity, stroke, heart disease, diabetes and cancer), and many other chronic problems associated with physical, emotional and behavioral strength and stability.

Today, less than ten cents of every grocery dollar is spent on fresh produce, while the food industry spends billions of dollars advertising foods that are not only deficient in nutrients, but are also seriously risky in the long-term effect they can have on our health and well-being.

More than 41 million Americans today have one or more forms of heart and blood vessel disease. Heart disease remains our number one killer. Obesity is also rampant, statistics suggesting that about eighty million Americans, or about forty percent of adults and approximately ten to fifteen percent of youngsters, are obese, and most of the latter are destined to become overweight adults. In addition to its cosmetic drawbacks, obesity is a risk factor in a number of leading health conditions.

According to the Senate Select Committee on Nutrition and Human Needs (1977), probably the most comprehensive assessment of America's dietary health, the dietary habits of Americans suggest many cases of borderline malnutrition.

The committee described our present pattern of both over- and underconsumption as being as profoundly damaging to the nation's health as the widespread contagious diseases of the early part of this century. They pointed out that foods high in fat, cholesterol, salt and sugar are connected with the major dietary health problems plaguing the nation.

Risks of Our Declining Diet

Senate Select Committee Recommendations

The nutrition experts who contributed to the Senate report proposed the following balance among fat, protein and carbohydrates (percentages refer to percent of total calorie needs):

FAT—30%
(10% saturated;
10% monounsaturated;
10% polyunsaturated)

PROTEIN—12%

CARBOHYDRATES—58%
(48% from naturally
occurring sugars and
complex carbohydrates;
10% from refined and
processed sugars)

Translation of recommendations for a moderately active teenage male or other person requiring about 3,000 calories per day:

		Calories Per Day			*Weight Per Day*
Saturated fat	10%	300	1 gram fat	= 9 calories	33 grams
Unsaturated fat	20%	600	1 gram fat	= 9 calories	66 grams
Protein	12%	360	1 gram protein	= 4 calories	90 grams
Complex carbohydrates	48%	1,440	1 gram carb.	= 4 calories	360 grams
Refined sugar	10%	300	1 gram sugar	= 4 calories	75 grams

Translation of recommendations for a moderately active teenage female or other person requiring about 2,100 calories per day:

		Calories Per Day			*Weight Per Day*
Saturated fat	10%	210	1 gram fat	= 9 calories	23 grams
Unsaturated fat	20%	420	1 gram fat	= 9 calories	47 grams
Protein	12%	252	1 gram protein	= 4 calories	63 grams
Complex carbohydrates	48%	1,008	1 gram carb.	= 4 calories	252 grams
Refined sugar	10%	210	1 gram sugar	= 4 calories	52 grams

NUTRITION AS BASIS OF GOOD HEALTH
Characteristics of a Well-Nourished Child

The well-nourished child may be expected to exhibit these characteristics:

Sense of well-being—Alert; interested in activities usual for the child's age; vigorous; happy
Vitality—Endurance during activity, quick recovery from fatigue; looks rested; does not fall asleep in school; sleeps well at night
Weight—Normal for height, age and body build
Posture—Erect; arms and legs straight; abdomen pulled in; chest out
Teeth—Straight, without crowding in well-shaped jaw
Gums—Firm, pink; no signs of bleeding
Skin—Smooth, slightly moist; healthy glow; reddish-pink mucous membranes
Eyes—Clear, bright; no circles of fatigue around them
Hair—Lustrous; healthy scalp
Muscles—Well developed; firm
Nervous control—Good attention span for the child's age; gets along well with others; does not cry easily; not irritable or restless
Gastrointestinal factors—good appetite; normal, regular elimination.

Source: *Normal and Therapeutic Nutrition*, 14th edition Corinne H. Robinson, MacMillan, 1982.

Food Factors Endangering Your Wellness

Sugars

The average American ingests about 125 pounds of sugar each year, most of which is hidden in canned, packaged and snack items. Many of these sugars are often disguised on the label with other names, but are included in the sugar group.

Beware—sugars can have many names:

sucrose	maltose
glucose	invert sugar
dextrose	raw sugar
corn sweetener	brown sugar
corn syrup	fructose
malt syrup	other syrups

Note: Mannitol is considered a "sugar-free" substitute, but has calories and carbohydrates (and may be linked to serious health conditions)

Keep in mind that food ingredients are listed on package labels in their order of quantity. This means ingredients listed at the beginning of labels are added

HOW SUGARS EASILY ADD UP
Some Samples

Sugary foods

1 tsp. jam or jelly	= 1 tsp. sugar, syrup or molasses
1-ounce chocolate bar	= 2 tsp. fat + 5 tsp. sugar
12 ounces fruit drink, ade or punch	= 12 tsp. sugar
12 ounces cola	= 9 tsp. sugar

Effects of Food Form and Preparation

½ cup frozen sweetened fruit	= ½ cup unsweetened fruit + 6 tsp. sugar
½ cup fruit, canned in heavy syrup	= ½ cup unsweetened fruit + 4 tsp. sugar
½ cup fruit, canned in light syrup	= ½ cup unsweetened fruit + 2 tsp. sugar
8 ounces low-fat vanilla-flavored yogurt	= 8 ounces low-fat milk + 4 tsp. sugar
8 ounces low-fat fruit yogurt	= 8 ounces low-fat milk + 7 tsp. sugar

Desserts

½ cup ice cream	= ⅓ cup skim milk + 2 tsp. fat + 3 tsp. sugar
½ cup ice milk	= ⅓ cup skim milk + 1 tsp. fat + 3 tsp. sugar
½ cup low-fat frozen yogurt	= ⅓ cup skim milk + 4 tsp. sugar
1/16 of white layer cake with chocolate frosting	= 1 slice bread + 3 tsp. fat + 6 tsp. sugar
2 oatmeal cookies	= 1 slice bread + 1 tsp. fat + 1 tsp. sugar
⅙ of 9-inch apple pie	= 2 slices bread + ⅓ medium apple + 3 tsp. fat + 6 tsp. sugar

Tradeoffs are approximations based on the calories and nutrients in these types of foods. Individual foods vary.

in greater percentage or proportions than those at the end of the ingredient list.

Some manufacturers attempt to confuse and mislead the public by listing four or five different kinds of sugar throughout the label. Since sugar isn't listed near the top of the label, the consumer, at first glance, may assume there isn't much sugar in the product—until he/she adds up all of the sugars on the label.

Fats and Cholesterol

Many Americans consume over fifty-five pounds of fats each year. Most of these fats are found, like sugar, hidden in our favorite treats. Presently, Americans have a fat consumption that accounts for about forty-five percent of our total calories. For good health, we need to lower fat consumption to no more than thirty percent of the total diet (and preferably lower). This includes all fats. Saturated fats, linked to high cholesterol, are found primarily in animal products (which are also high in cholesterol). These include eggs, dairy products and meat, and—in lesser quantity—poultry and fish. Keep in mind that coconut, palm, cottonseed and cocoabutter oils are also proportionately saturated. "Hydrogenated oils" are similar to, and often worse than, saturated fats in their effect on the body; thus, beware of margarine, vegetable shortenings, nondairy creamers and whipped toppings, all of which are often highly hydrogenated. High-heat oil, as used in preparing fast foods and most fried foods, can also be harmful to health. Research indicates that too much of any one type of fat can be harmful, yet, if we have a little bit of each (preferably in equal proportions of about ten percent each toward total of no more than thirty percent calories from fat), it is most sensible. Polyunsaturated and monounsaturated oils have been

Approximate Fat and Oil Breakdowns in Percentages

	Saturated	Monosaturated	Polyunsaturated
Butter	66.0	30.0	4.0
Corn Oil	14.5	27.6	57.9
Olive Oil	17.1	72.3	10.6
Peanut Oil	20.4	48.1	31.5
Safflower Oil	9.2	13.1	77.7
Soy Oil	15.6	23.4	61.0

touted as being the beneficial agents for reducing harmful blood cholesterol. More recently we see that monounsaturates may lead the way, since they seem to lower only harmful low-density lipoproteins (LDL—bad cholesterol), while allowing the high-density lipoproteins (HDL—good cholesterol) to remain fairly constant. Polyunsaturates also lower cholesterol levels, yet seem to fail to make the distinction between LDL and HDL, lowering both.

Are you aware of the percentage of fat calories in the foods you eat? Let's take a look!

Seventy-five percent or more—
   Avocado, olives, cold cuts and luncheon meats, peanuts and peanut butters, nuts and seeds, salt pork, cream cheese, creams, coconut, bacon, beef (chuck rib, sirloin, hamburger [regular], loin [untrimmed]), headcheese, frankfurters.

Fifty percent to seventy-five percent—
   Beef (rump and corned), Canadian bacon, cheeses (American, Swiss, bleu, cheddar) cream soups, eggs, ice cream (rich), fried oysters, tuna in oil and tuna salad, veal.

Food Factors Endangering Wellness

What's in Fast Foods?

Item	Calories	Protein (g)	Carbo-hydrates (g)	Fats (g)	Sodium (mg)
Burger King Whaler	486	18	64	46	735
Burger King Whopper	606	29	51	32	909
Dairy Queen Banana Split	540	10	91	15	NA*
Dairy Queen Onion Rings	300	6	33	17	NA
Kentucky Fried Chicken Extra Crispy Dinner (3 pieces chicken)	950	52	63	54	1,915
Long John Silver's Fish (2 pieces)	318	19	19	19	NA
McDonald's Big Mac	541	26	39	31	962
McDonald's Chocolate Shake	364	11	60	9	329
McDonald's Egg McMuffin	352	18	26	20	914
Pizza Hut Thin 'n Crispy Cheese Pizza (½ of 10-inch pie)	450	25	54	15	NA
Taco Bell Taco	186	15	14	8	79

Source: Data supplied by the companies to the Senate Select Committee on Nutrition and Human Needs.

*NA = Not available.

Forty percent to fifty percent—
  Lean hamburger, T-bone steak, fried chicken, regular ice cream, whole milk, whole-milk yogurt, canned salmon, drained sardines

Thirty percent to forty percent—
  Pot roast, flank steak, roasted chicken without skin, flounder, haddock (broiled), ice milk, two-percent

milk, tuna with drained oil, dark meat of turkey, low-fat yogurt

Twenty percent to thirty percent—
Pancakes, tomato and chicken noodle soup, wheat germ, corn muffin, raw oysters, lean sirloin beef

Less than twenty percent—
Beans, bread, cereals, uncreamed cottage cheese, fruits, grains, skim milk, consommé, split pea soups, tuna packed in water, white meat of turkey.

According to the latest American Heart Association guidelines, dietary cholesterol consumption is also a major consideration in reducing our risk for coronary heart disease. They remind us that we should limit daily cholesterol intake to no more than one hundred milligrams per one thousand calories and to no more than three hundred mg. daily. Considering that many foods are high in cholesterol, it is often easy to go above common guidelines.

Let's look at some typical cholesterol levels in foods. Remember, cholesterol is different from fat calories!

Cholesterol Levels

Food	Amount	Cholesterol (mg.)
Frankfurter	2 (4 oz. each)	112
Beef liver	3 oz.	372
Egg (white and yolk)	1 large	252
Chicken or turkey (white meat—without skin)	3 oz.	65
Turkey, dark (no skin)	3 oz.	86
Crab, canned	3 oz.	85
Shrimp, canned	3 oz.	128
Butter	1 tbsp.	35

Food Factors Endangering Wellness

Food	Amount	Cholesterol (mg.)
Cheese (hard)	1 oz.	24–28
1% cottage cheese	½ cup	12
Muffin, plain	3-inch diameter	21
Flounder	3 oz.	69
Veal	3 oz.	84
Lamb (lean)	3 oz.	85
Cornbread	1 oz.	58
Low-fat yogurt	1 cup	17

All foods from animal sources contain some cholesterol, and, of course, not everyone has a cholesterol problem. We cannot remain healthy without cholesterol. If we do not get sufficient amounts from our food, roughly two grams daily, the body simply makes that amount. A very low cholesterol level may contribute to some cancers.

Blood Cholesterol Guidelines for Children and Adults—1986

—How's Your Risk?

Age	Moderate Risk	High Risk
2–19	170–185 mg.	Above 185 mg.
20–29	200–220 mg.	Above 220 mg.
30–39	220–240 mg.	Above 240 mg.
40 and over	240–260 mg.	Above 260 mg.

Measured in milligrams (mg.) of cholesterol per deciliter of blood.

Source: American Heart Association and National Lung and Blood Institutes.

Sodium (Salt)

Salt is found primarily in commercially prepared foods, including most canned, packaged, convenience and snack items. It's also found in significant quantities in condiments and in many food additives. Without awareness, you can easily go many times over the maximum recommended levels of one thousand to three thousand milligrams daily.

Excess salts not only create potassium loss and water retention, but are also a factor in high blood pressure (along with, in many cases, obesity, high cholesterol, lack of exercise and smoking).

Normal Ranges of Blood Pressure

Blood pressure is always expressed in two numbers, which are measurements of millimeters of mercury (mm Hg) or an equivalent. For example:

$$\frac{120}{80} \text{ mm Hg} \quad \begin{array}{l} \text{systolic (pumping pressure)} \\ \text{diastolic (resting pressure)} \end{array}$$

Blood Pressure (mm Hg)

Age	Men	Women
19–29	100/70 to 130/80	100/70 to 120/80
30–49	130/85 to 135/85	125/80 to 130/85
50–69	140/90 to 145/90	135/85 to 150/90
70–	150/85	160/85

Regardless of age, the risk of cardiovascular complications increases as blood pressure rises above 135/85. As you get older, both systolic and diastolic values tend to increase progressively.

Food Factors Endangering Wellness
How Salt Adds Up

Salt–Sodium Conversions:
¼ tsp. salt = 500 mg. sodium
½ tsp. salt = 1,000 mg. sodium
¾ tsp. salt = 1,500 mg. sodium
1 tsp. salt = 2,000 mg. sodium

Common High-Sodium Food Items

White flour, self-rising
Canned vegetables
Canned fish
Hot dogs
Corned meats
Sauerkraut
Cheese
Bouillon
Baking soda
Onion, garlic, celery or seasoning
MSG (monosodium glutamate)
Soy sauce or tamari
Pickles
Relish
Chili sauce
Fried and breaded chicken
Catsup
Mustard
Worcestershire sauce
Salad dressings
Meat tenderizer
Barbecue sauce
Fast foods
TV dinners
Potato chips
Pretzels
Snack items (chips, dips)

Common Sodium Food Additives

Baking powder (leavening agent)
Baking soda (leavening agent)
Monosodium glutamate (flavor enhancer)
Sodium benzoate (preservative)
Sodium caseinate (thickener and binder)
Sodium citrate (buffer, used to control acidity in soft drinks and fruit drinks)

NUTRITION AS BASIS OF GOOD HEALTH

Sodium nitrite (curing agent in meat, provides color, prevents botulism)
Sodium phosphate (emulsifier, stabilizer, buffer)
Sodium propionate (mold inhibitor)
Sodium saccharin (artificial sweetener)

Healthier Alternatives:
How to Season Your Food Without Salt*

Meat, Fish and Poultry

Beef	Bay leaf, dry mustard powder, green pepper, marjoram, fresh mushrooms, nutmeg, onion, pepper, sage, thyme.
Chicken	Green pepper, lemon juice, marjoram, fresh mushrooms, paprika, parsley, sage, thyme.
Fish	Bay leaf, curry powder, dry mustard powder, green pepper, lemon juice, marjoram, fresh mushrooms, paprika.
Lamb	Curry powder, garlic, mint, mint jelly, pineapple, rosemary.
Pork	Apple, applesauce, garlic, onion, sage.
Veal	Apricot, bay leaf, curry powder, ginger, marjoram, oregano.

Vegetables

Asparagus	Garlic, lemon juice, onion, vinegar.
Corn	Green pepper, pimiento, fresh tomato.
Cucumbers	Chives, dill, garlic, vinegar.
Green beans	Dill, lemon juice, marjoram, nutmeg, pimiento.
Greens	Onion, pepper, vinegar.
Peas	Green pepper, mint, fresh mushrooms, onion, parsley.
Potatoes	Green pepper, mace, onion, paprika, parsley.
Rice	Chives, green pepper, onion, pimiento, saffron.

---

*From *Cooking Without Your Salt Shaker,* by the American Heart Association (available for purchase from local chapters).

Food Factors Endangering Wellness

Squash	Brown sugar, cinnamon, ginger, mace, nutmeg, onion.
Tomatoes	Basil, marjoram, onion, oregano.

Soups

Bean	Pinch of dry mustard powder.
Milk Chowders	Peppercorns.
Pea	Bay leaf and parsley.
Vegtable	Vinegar, dash of sugar.

Food Additives

Chemical preservatives, artificial colors, sweeteners, stabilizers, emulsifiers and other troublesome or potentially toxic substances commonly fall into the category of food additives. The vast majority of commercial, packaged and processed foods contain a tremendous assortment of hidden additives. Our favorite snacks, luncheon meats, canned, frozen and prepared food products are often sources of overwhelming numbers of chemicals that can create many serious health problems. Currently, most European countries seem far more aware and concerned about food purity; they use only a small amount of additives. We, in the U.S., however, are commonly bombarded with a tremendous assortment of chemical substances. Besides the harmful effects identified with substances such as caffeine, sugar and BHA/BHT, American foods, drugs and cosmetics contain many of the following substances linked to allergies or to various forms of cancer, tumors or chromosomal damage.

Additive Avoidance

FD&C red 3
FD&C yellow 5
FD&C yellow 6

D&C red 8
D&C red 9

D&C red 33
D&C orange 17
D&C red 19
D&C red 37
D&C red 36

7 Remaining U.S. Food Dyes

Avoid:

Red 3
Red 40
Blue 1
Blue 2

Green 3
Yellow 5
Yellow 6

Other Additives and Their Risks

- Artificial colors (allergies) citrus red 2
- BHA/BHT (cancer)
- Caffeine
- Monosodium glutamate
- Propyl gallate (cancer)
- Saccharin (cancer)
- Quinine
- Sodium nitrite (cancer)
- Sulfiting agents (asthma/allergies)

Toxic Metals

Toxic metals, the residues of which are often absorbed into our bodies, can create serious physical, mental, muscular and neurological impairments. These substances can sneak into our diet through lead-sealed

Food Factors Endangering Wellness

cans, fish from industrial or polluted waters, tap water, copper, or soldered piping, utensils and, often, through added metals (*i.e.*, aluminum in antacids and cookware; cadmium in coffee) used in foods. There are other sources of such exposure as well.

Potential Human Exposures to Toxic Trace Metals

Metal or Element	Source of Exposure
	Toxic
Antimony	Pewter, britannia metal, rubber, flameproof textiles, dyes, paint, ceramics, type metal, medicines
Arsenic	Insecticides, fungicides, weed killers, majolica (earthenware), alloys, medicines, pigments
Beryllium	Copper alloys, ceramics, rocket fuels
Cadmium	Plating, alloys, pigments, insecticides, solders, cigarette smoke, plastics, rubber, galvanized iron
Lead	Tetraethyl lead in gasoline (largest use), pipes, cisterns, paint, alloys, solders, glass, pottery glazes, rubber, plastics, insecticides, pewter
Mercury	Paint, solders, fungistates, amalgams, drugs, disinfectants, jewelry Organic mercury in seed dressings, paint
	Slightly Toxic
Barium	Alloys, paints, rubber, soap, linoleum, sugar, ceramics, insecticides, paper
Bismuth	Pharmaceuticals, alloys
Gallium	Alloys, glass-sealing compound
Germanium	Electroplating, alloys, catalyst for hydrogenation of coal
Lanthanum	Lighter flints, weighting of silk and rayon
Nickel	Alloys, steels, coins, enamels, ceramics, glass, catalyst for hydrogenation of oils
Rhodium	Alloys, jewelry, plating

NUTRITION AS BASIS OF GOOD HEALTH

Tin	Tin plate, alloys, collapsible tubes, foil, plastics, rubber, fungicides, insecticides, drugs, toothpaste
Tungsten	Alloys, plating, flameproofing of cloth, pigments
Zirconium	Alloys, lighter flints, ceramics, pigment, plastics, catalyst, antiperspirants

Source: *The Poisons Around Us,* H. Schroeder, Keats Publishing, Inc., 1974.

Overprocessed and Overcooked Foods

Canned, packaged, boxed, frozen foodlike (imitation) products, ready-to-eat, and food items stored for prolonged periods can create less than optimal nutrition

Nutrients Lost in Refining Whole Products

Percentages lost in refinement of whole raw wheat, raw sugar, unpolished rice, whole corn and whole milk.

Nutrient	Wheat flour	Sugar, refined	Rice, polished	Corn starch	Milk, fat-free
Ash	76	88	—	—	32
Calcium	60	—	—	—	—
Chromium	40	93	75	72	>50
Cobalt	89	95	38	37	0
Copper	68	83	26	31	0
Iron	76	—	—	—	—
Magnesium	85	98	83	97	6
Manganese	86	89	45	93	100
Molybdenum	48	100	—	—	90
Phosphorus	71	—	—	—	—
Selenium	16	100	—	100	88
Strontium	95	96	—	—	0
Vitamin B_6	72	100	69	87	—
Zinc	78	98	75	91	14

Source: *The Poisons Around Us,* H. Schroeder, Keats Publishing, Inc., 1974.

Food Factors Endangering Wellness

levels. They also provide us with too many negative health-risk factors. Excessive cooking can also deprive our bodies of the nourishment nature intended in the food. Organic foods offer the extra benefit of purity, plus soil-enriched foods generally have higher nutrient ranges.

Suggested Cooking Methods
(To retain maximum nutrients)

Vegetables
- Quick steam
- Quick boil
- Light sauté (oil or water)
- Blanch
- Light stir-fry
- Pressure-cook

Grains/Beans/Legumes
- Boil
- Pressure-cook
- Crock pot

Leftovers
- Steam
- Stir-fry

Avoid deep frying and steaming or boiling vegetables to the point of losing crispness or color.

Insecticide-Treated or Irradiated Foods

Thorough cleaning of all market produce with a firm, natural bristle brush provides some protection against harmful residues of fumigants and insecticides. Scraping and peeling skins of fruits and vegetables are other important considerations to avoid exposure.

Irradiated products can be a big health threat. Read labels carefully to avoid these treated products. Irradiation, a process believed to reduce spoilage, kill pests and eliminate bacteria, is under serious investigation by many independent research groups. New findings regarding the hazards of irradiation are gaining much attention. They find that irradiation will not eliminate hazardous pesticides (*i.e.*, fumigants, ethylene dibromide [EDB], etc. used on various commodities), nor will it necessarily control trichinosis in pork products; yet it can create potentially carcinogenic by-products in treated foods. These by-products could potentially damage blood, kidneys and other body organs and tissues.

New food irradiation safety and labeling bills calling for more research are being introduced in many states. Without passage of many of these bills, consumers will not be able to avoid irradiated foods. Already, one percent of spices are irradiated and used in processed foods without notation on the label. It's impossible to tell if your slice of prepared pizza, for example, has irradiated spices in its sauce. In Japan, for example, some potatoes are irradiated to prevent sprouting but are not labeled and are not sold directly to the public. Such potatoes are, however, used in processed food and restaurant foods. In England and West Germany, irradiation remains banned.

Currently, the FDA has approved irradiation of fruits, vegetables, pork, grain, potatoes, spices and seasonings, but as of this writing only spices and some prepared foods are routinely being irradiated.

Food Factors Endangering Wellness

Foods Approved for Irradiation

Food	Dose	Effect
Fresh fruits and vegetables	100,000 rads*	Kills insects, inhibits sprouting and ripening, extends shelf life by killing bacteria and retarding some mold development.
Pork	100,000 rads	Sterilizes trichina larvae, the organism that causes trichinosis; extends shelf life by killing bacteria.
Wheat and wheat flour	100,000 rads	Kills insects, retards some mold development
Some spices, such as anise, caraway seed, chives, etc.	3,000,000 rads	Kills insects, extends shelf life by killing bacteria
Dried enzyme preparations (*e.g.*, meat tenderizer)	3,000,000 rads	Extends shelf life by killing bacteria

*A rad is the unit by which radiation doses are measured.
Source: Food and Drug Administration.

Caffeine

Although some medications (such as those commonly prescribed for migraine and pain relief) depend upon caffeine for their effectiveness, excess caffeine can create a broad array of health difficulties. We know, for example, that a cup of morning java can perk up your brain, but when we keep going back for more we can be inviting trouble. Of special concern are hyperactive children, who often get "hard to handle" because of large amounts of caffeine stimulants in their diet in colas, chocolates, cocoa and some medications.

The Effects of Caffeine

Caffeine can
1. irritate the gastrointestinal tract
2. be taxing to the liver
3. cause ringing in your ears
4. cause headaches
5. cause anxiety and aggravate stress and tension
6. cause nervousness
7. give you a lift but will drop you down lower than you were
8. create an addiction
9. dehydrate you because of increased urination
10. cause hyperactivity
11. make your heart beat faster
12. create vitamin and mineral losses
13. be associated with heart attacks and elevated blood fats
14. cause indigestion, peptic ulcers
15. cause heartburn
16. cause muscle tension
17. cause trouble falling asleep
18. damage a developing fetus
19. have a negative effect on the mind and mood
20. create blood sugar fluctuations.

Food Factors Endangering Wellness

Approximate Caffeine Content of Common Beverages*

Coffee (brewed)	100–110 mg./6-oz. serving
Coffee (instant)	70–75 mg./6-oz. serving
Coffee (decaffeinated)	3–5 mg./6-oz. serving
Tea (instant)	30–36 mg./6-oz. serving
Tea (brewed)	50–100 mg./6-oz. serving
Cola beverages	36–65 mg./12-oz. serving
Cocoa	6–142 mg./5-oz. serving
Chocolate	20 mg./1-oz. serving

*Sources: Johns Hopkins Hospital Dietary Manual (1973); Stephenson (1977); Massachusetts General Hospital Dietary Manual (1976).

Also note that caffeine is commonly found in these nonprescription drugs:

- weight control aids (high amounts)
- alertness tablets
- analgesic/pain relief
- diuretics (high amounts)
- cold/allergy remedies

Tap Water

Increasing evidence indicating high levels of pollution in our public water supplies as well as oceans, lakes and streams forces us to reconsider the quality of our beverages and the purity of the fish we consume. Greater awareness is being focused on the many toxic substances found in these waters since EPA standards and testing are often ineffective. High amounts of chlorine, chlorinated hydrocarbons, softeners, lead, copper, cadmium and other industrial chemicals, cancer-causing chloroform, trihalmethanes and other hidden and identifiable substances are commonly found. It is not uncommon for public drinking waters to contain thousands of identifiable (and unidentifiable) chemicals and substances that may be hazardous to our health. An alternative is to use a highly rated carbon filter water system, to avoid drinking water that has been softened or to purchase spring or distilled water as a healthier substitute. Distilled water, of course, has had all minerals—including beneficial ones—removed.

Water is often considered our number one nutritional deficiency. Few people realize how important water is to our health, and thus often fail to drink sufficient amounts of water (six to eight glasses, or about one eight-ounce glass for each twenty-five pounds of body weight, every day). Drinking soda, juice, hot beverages and soup should be an addition to our water intake and not our major source of water.

Alcohol

In moderation (less than two ounces daily), alcohol is generally considered to be safe for adults and women who are not pregnant. Yet, in excess, alcohol can create many hazardous physical and psychological dependencies:

Liver Damage—especially cirrhosis (scarring of the liver), fat accumulation in the liver, alcoholic hepatitis and liver cancer.

Heart Disease—including enlarged heart, congestive heart failure, hypertension, lowered cardiovascular endurance and cardiomyopathy, an unexplained heart muscle disease

Ulcers and Gastritis—due to irritation of the stomach lining by alcohol and increased secretion of gastric acids

Malnutrition—alcohol not only interferes with digestion, but excess amounts can also create a loss of important vitamins and minerals

Cancer—risks are increased, especially to the mouth, breast, stomach and esophagus

Brain Damage—alcohol can cause a loss of brain cells, possible atrophy and psychosis

Damage to Developing Fetus—if a mother drinks alcohol during pregnancy, it can alter the cell structure.

For everyday understanding, most tolerance scales use a "per drink" standard to determine blood alcohol content, or percentage in relation to sex and body weight. Generally, the body can deal with about one drink every one and a half hours, but this can take longer for smaller people. About ninety percent of this is metabolized, or broken down, in the liver, and a small percent is lost in the urine, sweat and breath.

The following drinks have approximately equal alcohol content:

- 12 ounces of beer
- 4 ounces of table wine (*or* 5 oz. of 12% wine)
- 1½ ounces of 80-proof whiskey
- 2½ ounces of sherry
- 1¼ ounces of 86-proof spirits
- 1 ounce of 100-proof spirits

NUTRITION AS BASIS OF GOOD HEALTH

The following tables show blood alcohol content (percent) in relation to sex, body weight, and the number of drinks consumed. NOTE: 0.10 is legal intoxication.

Men

Body weight in pounds	1	2	3	4	5	6	7	8
100	0.04	0.09	0.13	0.16	0.22	0.26	0.30	0.35
120	0.04	0.07	0.11	0.14	0.18	0.22	0.25	0.29
140	0.03	0.06	0.09	0.12	0.16	0.19	0.22	0.28
160	0.03	0.05	0.08	0.11	0.14	0.16	0.19	0.22
180	0.02	0.05	0.07	0.10	0.12	0.14	0.17	0.20
200	0.02	0.04	0.06	0.09	0.11	0.13	0.15	0.17
220	0.02	0.04	0.06	0.08	0.10	0.12	0.14	0.16
240	0.02	0.04	0.06	0.07	0.09	0.10	0.12	0.14
260	0.02	0.03	0.05	0.07	0.08	0.10	0.12	0.13

Women

Body weight in pounds	1	2	3	4	5	6	7	8
80	0.06	0.12	0.18	0.25	0.31	0.37	—	—
100	0.05	0.10	0.15	0.22	0.25	0.29	0.34	0.39
120	0.04	0.08	0.12	0.17	0.21	0.25	0.29	0.33
140	0.04	0.07	0.11	0.14	0.18	0.21	0.25	0.28
160	0.03	0.06	0.09	0.12	0.15	0.19	0.22	0.25
180	0.03	0.06	0.08	0.11	0.14	0.15	0.19	0.22
200	0.02	0.05	0.07	0.10	0.12	0.15	0.17	0.20

Source: Carolina Biological Supply, Burlington, NC 27215, "What About Alcohol."

The Alcohol Abuse Interest Group says that for a healthy 150-pound inexperienced drinker, quickly con-

Food Factors Endangering Wellness

suming alcohol on an empty stomach can create these effects:

Drinks	Effect	Blood Alcohol Level
1	Slight feeling changes	0.03%
2	Mental relaxation	0.06%
3	Exaggerated emotions, excitement	0.09%
4	Clumsiness, slurring words, forgetfulness	0.12%

Legal intoxication for most states is .10 percent. At this level of intoxication:

- Eyes don't focus or track objects well
- Night and peripheral vision are reduced
- Reflex and reaction time is slower
- Judgment is impaired
- Inhibitions are lessened
- Risk behavior increases
- Normal integrated actions and movements become less coordinated.

Above this level, the drinker may obviously appear drunk to a nondrinker, yet the drinker is unaware of his impairments and may generally even feel capable of top performance.

Higher amounts of alcohol would generally create the following conditions for the same 150-pound individual:

Drinks	Effect	Blood Alcohol Level
10	Stuporous, deep sleep	0.30%
13	Coma, slowed breathing	0.40%
16	Death	0.50%

NUTRITION AS BASIS OF GOOD HEALTH
Sensitivities and Allergies

Avoiding foods and substances that provoke negative reactions is not only helpful to our physical and mental ease and comfort, such steps can also help to protect our bodies from potentially harmful reactions and the long-range damage these reactions may do to our immune system. Diet surveys, allergy and other biochemical, psychological, and cognitive tests and surveys can help pinpoint environmental and food sensitivities and allergies, and the reactions they are creating.

Besides seasonal and weather-related difficulties—such as pollen, ragweed, mold and other reactions—many people demonstrate subtle to very profound reactions to particular industrial, commercial and environmental chemicals (*i.e.*, dyes, inks, fumes, auto exhaust, clothing and fabric treatments), bee stings, common foods and food colors and additives. Among the most prevalent are the yeast- and mold-related substances, sulfites and even certain foods.

Milk and other dairy products, wheat, corn, sugar, eggs, yeast, soy and citrus are often among the most frequently cited food sensitivities. Salicylates, a group of naturally occurring food substances identified by Dr. Benjamin Feingold, also seem to play a role in hyperactivity and similar reactions associated with behavioral, cognitive/perceptual, skeletal/muscular, neurological, gastrointestinal, skin, ear and respiratory-related difficulties occurring quite commonly in children. Dr. Feingold first removed children (and adults) from all foods containing artificial (synthetic) colors and flavors (BHA, BHT and TBHQ). If no relief was found, he suggested the elimination of foods containing natural salicylates in all forms—fresh, frozen, canned, dried, as juice or as an ingredient in prepared food.

Food Factors Endangering Wellness

Naturally Occurring Salicylates
(second stage of avoidance testing)

Fruits—Almonds, apples (and cider and cider vinegar), apricots, berries—blackberries, boysenberries, gooseberries, raspberries, strawberries—cherries, currants, grapes and raisins or any product made from grapes (*e.g.*, wine, wine vinegar, jellies), nectarines, oranges, peaches, plums, prunes

Vegetables—Tomatoes (all tomato products), cucumbers, pickles, green peppers (and chilies)

Other—Coffee, cloves, oil of wintergreen (methylsalicylate).

Any natural or synthetically made food or substance can provoke a reaction, but what is often quite helpful is for allergy-sensitive individuals to be aware of interrelated foods and foods in related families that can induce any number of reactions. Since allergies are often subtle and baffling enough to have earned the epithet of "the great masquerader," such awareness is often crucial in ensuring your health.

Allergies are not always inherited, but tendencies and susceptibilities are. Thus, if one parent is allergic to certain agents, chances are about fifty percent that a child will also be allergic. If both parents are, the odds jump to seventy-five percent.

Understanding Allergies

Allergies are an overreaction of the immune system to an agent that the body interprets as harmful. Normally, our immune system will recognize and destroy these harmful agents or foreign invaders. It does this by releasing natural antibodies. After fighting, some cells remain in the lymph as "memory" in case the invaders (antigens) they fought invade the body again. These antibody memory cells gradually desensitize cells. Often, for some unknown reason, they perceive some of the otherwise harmless substances (such as milk, wheat or corn) as an enemy antigen. When these enemy allergens are encountered, the cells release natural substances called histamines. Sometimes, however, excess histamines are produced, causing blood vessel inflammation and other signs and symptoms of a reactive response. Your physician may suggest avoidance of the offending substance, plus a regime of steps to counteract the body's response. This will generally include avoidance of the substances and diet rotation, immune bolstering with special supplements, stress management and lifestyle changes, plus, in some cases, neutralization therapy.

Common Symptoms of Allergy Response in Children and Adults

- Dark circles ("allergic shiners") or puffiness under eyes
- Headache, some migraine
- Dizziness
- Bouts of sneezing
- Coughing when laughing or exercising
- Canker sores
- Diarrhea
- Rubbing the nose upward (especially seen in children)
- Itching skin
- Irregular menstruation
- Sensitivity to light, sound or cold
- Poor appetite
- Excessive perspiration
- Pale, sallow look
- Frequent or persistent colds
- Stomachache
- Low-grade fever
- Numbness or tingling
- Violent outbreaks
- Gastrointestinal problems
- Jock itch
- Constipation
- Visual problems
- Vaginal discharge (especially yeast and Candida related)
- Premenstrual syndrome (PMS)
- Increased tendency to react to moldy, damp or muggy places

Food Factors Endangering Wellness

- Restlessness, insomnia
- Excessive throat mucus
- Excessive bowel mucus
- Excessive drooling
- Muscle aches
- Joint aches or swelling
- Bed-wetting
- Frequent urination
- Swollen hands, feet, face
- Tender, sore skin and skin rashes
- Tiredness after naps or eating
- Irritability
- Depression
- Behavior problems and hyperactivity
- Clucking throat sounds
- Mottled tongue
- Sudden weight gain (5 pounds or more in one or two days)
- Fatigue
- Inability to concentrate
- Addictivelike cravings
- Kick-drop response to food or drink
- Sleep problems
- Glazed eyes
- Increased sensitivity to smoke and fumes or scents
- Chronic fungal infections (feet, hands, nails)
- Recurrent ringworm

Common Food Families

NOTE: You may show cross-sensitivity to foods within the same family.

Banana
Banana
Beech
Chestnuts
Bellflower, Thistle
Artichoke
Lettuce
Safflower oil
Sunflower oil
Birch
Filbert
Bony Fish
Bass
Catfish
Cod
Flounder
Halibut
Herring
Mackerel
Mullet
Perch
Red snapper
Salmon
Sardine
Smelt
Sole
Swordfish
Trout
Tuna
Brassica
Broccoli
Brussels sprouts
Cabbage
Cauliflower
Kale
Radish
Turnip
Buckthorn
Grape, raisin
Buckwheat
Buckwheat
Rhubarb
Carica
Papaya
Carrot
Caraway
Carrot
Celery

NUTRITION AS BASIS OF GOOD HEALTH

Parsnip
Cartilaginous fish
Shark
Cashew
Cashew
Mango
Cereal grains (grasses)
Barley
Cane sugar
Corn (maize)
Corn sugar
Hops
Malt
Millet
Oats
Rice
Rye
Wheat
Wild rice
Composite
Endive
Crustaceans
Crab
Lobster
Shrimp
Cyperaceae
Water chestnuts
Farinosa
Pineapple
Fungus
Baker's yeast
Brewer's yeast
Mushroom
Ginger
Ginger
Turmeric
Gourd Order
Cantaloupe
Cranshaw melon
Cucumber
Honeydew melon
Pumpkin
Squash (summer)
Squash (winter)
Watermelon
Heath
Blueberry
Boysenberry
Gooseberry
Honeysuckle
Cranberry
Laurel
Avocado
Cinnamon
Legume
Alfalfa
Bean (kidney)
Bean (lima)
Bean (mung)
Bean (pinto)
Bean (soy)
Bean (string)
Black-eyed pea
Carob
Chickpea (garbanzo)
Lentil
Pea
Peanut
Split pea
Lily
Asparagus
Chives
Garlic
Leek
Onion
Madder
Coffee
Mallow
Cottonseed
Mammals
Beef
Butter
Calf's liver
Cheese (American)
Cheese (bleu)
Cheese (cottage)
Cheese (mozzarella)
Cheese (parmesan)
Cheese (Swiss)
Cow's milk
Lamb
Pork
Yogurt
Maple
Maple sugar
Mollusks
Abalone
Clam
Oyster
Mulberry
Fig
Mustard
Collard greens
Mustard
Myristiceae
Nutmeg (mace)
Myrtle
Clove
Nightshade
Eggplant
Chili pepper
Garden peppers
Paprika
Potato
Tobacco
Tomato
Nightshade—Mint
Peppermint (spearmint)
Sage

Food Factors Endangering Wellness

Nightshade—
Morning Glory
Sweet potato
(maroon) yam
Sweet potato
(yellow)
Nightshade—
Pedalium
Sesame
Orchid
Vanilla
Palm
Date
Coconut
Parsley
Watercress
Pepper
Black pepper
Pink
Beet
Beet sugar
Spinach
Swiss chard
Poultry
Chicken

Chicken egg white
Chicken egg yolk
Duck
Goose
Pheasant
Turkey
Rose
Apple
Apricot
Blackberry
Cherry (prunus)
Nectarine
Peach
Pear
Plum, prune
Strawberry
Rue
Grapefruit
Lemon
Lime
Orange
Tangerine
Sapucaia
Brazil nut

Spurgel
Curry
Tapioca, cassava,
yucca
Sterculia
Cocoa, chocolate
Cola nut
Tea
Pecan
Tea, black
Walnut
Other
Allspice
Almond
Aspirin
Food coloring
Goat's milk
Honey
Horseradish
MSG
Olives
Oregano
Saccharin
Thyme

Foods Containing Yeast
(a major allergy substance)

Breads
Crackers
Pastries
Pretzels
Hamburger and
hot dog buns
Cake and cake mix
Cookies
Flour enriched with vitamins from
yeast
Rolls, homemade and canned
Canned ice box cookies and biscuits
Milk fortified with vitamins from
yeast
Meat or fish fried in cracker crumbs

NUTRITION AS BASIS OF GOOD HEALTH

Other yeast-containing foods or yeast-like substances because of their nature or their manufacture or preparation:

Antibiotics
Mushrooms
Truffles
Cheese of all kinds (except fresh)
Buttermilk
Cottage cheese
Vinegar:
  apple
  gin
  pear
  grape
  distilled
Catsup
Mayonnaise
Olives
Pickles
Sauerkraut
Condiments
Horseradish
French dressing
Salad dressing
Barbecue sauce
Sour cream
Citric acid
Dried and cured foods
Teas
Peanuts
Tomato sauce
Chili peppers
Mince pie
Gerber's oatmeal
Barley cereal
Alcoholic beverages:
  whiskey
  beer
  wine
  brandy
  rum
  vodka
Root beer
Malted products:
  cereals
  candy
  malted milk drinks
Frozen or canned citrus fruit and juices
Vitamin products (many are derived from yeast or have their sources from yeast [especially B-complex])
Dried fruits
Fermented beverages
Soy sauce, tamari
Smoked foods
Dried roasted nuts

NOTE: Yeast problems (candidiasis or *Candida albicans*) are often aggravated by sugary foods and carbohydrate-rich diets.

Food Factors Endangering Wellness

Special Alert for Asthmatics and the Sulfite-sensitive

Many foods ordinarily considered healthful may not be good choices for sulfite-sensitive or sulfite-allergic–prone individuals.

According to studies by Dr. D. Edward Buckley, Professor of Allergy and Respiratory Diseases at Duke University, more than 400,000 Americans experience adverse reactions to sulfites. Additionally, of the more than ten million asthmatics in the US estimates find more than 460,000 sensitive to sulfites.

Adverse reactions to sulfites range from nausea, hives, diarrhea, flushing, faintness, weakness, tongue swelling, difficulty swallowing or breathing, chest tightness, serious allergic reactions such as shock, acute asthma and loss of consiousness.

In August 1985, the FDA concluded that the use of sulfites on fruits and vegetables is no longer to be considered GRAS (generally recognized as safe). They also proposed a ban on their use. As a new requirement, the FDA will now be requiring that a sulfite "warning" be placed on prescription drugs. There are presently more than 1,100 oxygen-sensitive prescription drugs containing sulfites! Most, however, are inhalants (bronchodilators) and drugs commonly used in standard medical practice. Some of these are often used by the asthmatic or other sulfite-sensitive populations.

Where do we look for sulfites?

- *Read Labels*. Words like sodium or potassium "metabisulfite," "bisulfite" and "sulfite" and "sulfurdioxide" are keys.

- *Ask Your Physician* about which prescribed drugs and medications contain sulfites.
- *Watch Your Diet*. Watch sulfite-sprayed salad bars; many wines; preservatives in bottled beer, fruit drinks, baked goods, dried fruit; shellfish; canned or dried soups and frozen, canned or dried potatoes—packaged and processed foods bought in most stores. Be aware that present labeling laws allow food producers to loophole, and leave out many of the ingredients. The FDA requires that sulfites be eliminated at salad bars, since several people have died from allergic reactions to these chemicals.

Major Foods with Possible Sulfites*

Avocado and guacamole dips
Beer, cider, wine, fruit juices
Fruits (prepared and dried), purées, fillings, relishes
Sauces, gravies, salad dressings, wine vinegar
Vegetables (pre-cut, canned, frozen and dried)
Shellfish (all, fresh and commercially prepared) and dried codfish
Gelatin
Soups (canned or dried)
Sauerkraut, coleslaw, fresh mushrooms
Potatoes (pre-cut and commercially prepared)

It's strongly advised to check for these substances in all other food, beverage and medication sources.

*Sources: Schiff Nutrition Alert, Vol. 2. No. 2. FDA (DHS) Nov. 20, 1985, Consumer Letter.

ESSENTIALS OF BASIC HEALTHFUL EATING

"The Undesirables"

The preceding section discussed in detail the various food factors most harmful to us—here's a handy summary list of what to shun to avoid intake of those factors.

1. Commercially processed flour products:
   white breads, white buns, biscuits, white rolls, egg noodles, crackers, cookies, cakes, doughnuts, spaghetti, macaroni, dumplings, pie crusts
2. Commercially processed white sugar (and artificially sweetened) products:
   candy, soda (all types), pie, pudding and other very fatty or sugary foods
3. If you are concerned about fat and cholesterol, all regular and high-fat dairy products (regular milk, light, heavy and sour cream, cheese products, ice cream)
4. All fried foods and fast foods
5. Chips, dips and greasy foods
6. All hydrogenated oils

7. Ground, processed meats (including smoked, cured and barbecued)
8. Canned, packed and prepared foods with additives, added sugars, salts and fats
9. Alcohol in excess.
10. Caffeine (especially in excess)

"The Desirables"

Sensible eating and more healthful living starts with your choices of how you live. We are subjected every day to stress factors in our environment and in our emotional or personal life. All stress, when mishandled, becomes distress—the negative factor that could alter our health and well-being. Our diet, too, can be stress-filled, especially when it contains harmful factors.

When possible, always purchase seasonal and local fruits and vegetables. Your next choice should be frozen products, while the last should be packaged or canned. Always read labels—watch out for sugars, fats (especially "hydrogenated oils and fats"), salts and chemicals! Include these produce choices daily in generous amounts and complement your meals with high-quality, low-fat proteins such as fresh fish and naturally raised (often called "organic") poultry, and occasional lean red meats (try wild game, it's very natural). Vegetarian proteins, as derived from properly combining whole grains, beans (legumes), nuts, seeds and low-fat dairy products, can also offer excellent low-fat, high-fiber and nutritionally healthful nutrients—plus they are very economical selections! If you are new to vegetarianism, read *Diet for a Small Planet* by Frances Moore Lappé to learn how to combine seeds, nuts and grains for complete protein.

Essentials of Basic Healthful Eating

Healthful Shopping List

Include:

SOUPS   Various broth stocks from vegetables, poultry, meats with added vegetables, pasta, beans or tofu. You may also use miso if sodium is not restricted.

VEGETABLES   *Green and White Leafy:* Bok choy, Boston, Bibb lettuces; carrot tops, Chinese cabbage; collard greens, daikon greens, dandelion greens, kale, mustard greens, turnip greens, spinach; parsley; scallions; leeks; watercress

Stem/Root: Burdock, carrots, daikon (long white radish), dandelion, lotus, okra, radish, rutabaga, jinenjo (mountain potato), turnips, parsnips

Ground: Cauliflower, acorn squash, broccoli, brussels sprouts, butternut squash, cabbage, hubbard squash, pumpkin, red cabbage, string beans

Others: Celery, chives, cucumber, endive, escarole, sprouts, mushrooms, romaine and iceburg lettuces, green peas, tomato, snow peas, snap beans, Jerusalem artichokes, water chestnuts, hearts of palm, mushrooms, Swiss chard, beets, bamboo shoots, potato, yams, asparagus, peppers, zucchini, avocado

FRUITS AND MELONS   Apples, strawberries, cherries, blueberries, watermelon, cantaloupe, bananas, pears, peaches, plums, raspberries, apricots, grapes, natural raisins, oranges, pineapples, grapefruits, papaya, figs.

NUTRITION AS BASIS OF GOOD HEALTH

WHOLE GRAINS AND CEREALS	Short- and long-grain brown rice, whole rye, buckwheat groats (Kasha), millet, oats (whole, rolled, cracked or steel-cut), wheat berries, bulgur, cracked wheat, corn, barley, couscous, triticale, oat bran, rice bran, wheat bran, nondairy wholegrain creamed cereals, wheat germ, unsweetened granola, puffed whole grains, mixed wholegrain cereals, oat cereals, mochi (pounded sweet brown rice)
NOODLES AND PASTAS	Japanese soba, udon, somen, noodles and pasta (artichoke, spinach, buckwheat and wholegrain), ramen unbleached
BREADS	Wholegrain unleavened and/or unyeasted breads, Essene (sprouted) breads, wholegrain pitas, wholegrain unsweetened rolls and muffins, sourdough breads, rice cakes, wholegrain crackers, rice breads, gluten-free breads
BEANS (LEGUMES)	Aduki, green lentils, garbanzo (chickpeas), black soybeans, black, fava, mung, marrow, soy, black-eyed, split peas, red, pink, pinto, navy, great northern (white), tofu (soybean curd), dried tofu, natto (whole cooked soybeans); with the exception of tempeh and peanuts, soak and cook all beans well
SEA VEGETABLES	Dulse (soups), kelp (garnish), nori (garnish), wakame (soups), hijiki (side dish), kombu (soups), arame (side dish), Irish moss (soups), mekabu (side dish)
NUTS, SEEDS AND OILS	Various raw or lightly roasted (best unsalted) nuts, such as: almonds, walnuts, pecans, chestnuts; and seeds such as: ses-

Essentials of Basic Healthful Eating

ame, pumpkin and sunflower; nutbutters, such as tahini and sesame butter, almond and cashew butter in addition to peanuts; natural cold-pressed vegetable oils and nut oils: olive oil (extra virgin is best), canola sesame oils, safflower, sunflower, corn, mixed, flaxseed (natural "edible" linseed), mustard seed oil

FRESH FISH Especially good are the white fleshy fish and those from deep seas: salmon, tuna, sole, flounder, halibut, haddock, carp, trout, red snapper, cod, fresh herring, smelt; others: mackerel, shrimp, scallops, Irko (small dried fish), lobster, oysters, clams. *Always try to be sure fish comes from clean, unpolluted waters.*

MEATS AND POULTRY Chicken, turkey, pheasant, quail, venison, veal, beef (organic or wild game preferred)

BEVERAGES Spring and purified waters, kukicha (Bancha) twig tea, Pau d'Arco tea, roasted barley, roasted rice and Kombu teas, grain beverages and herbal teas (nonmedicinal)

CONDIMENTS AND SALAD STUFFS Tamari and tamari light, miso, sea salt, light salt, salt-free substitutes, fresh assorted herbs, natural mustards and catsups, ginger and natural dressings, umaboshi plums, gamashio and tekka (root) condiments

SNACKS AND EXTRA STAPLES Natural vinegars (apple cider, rice, grain, umaboshi), popcorn (air-popped), whole grain and vegetable crackers, puffed grains, unsweetened carob (chocolate substitute) powder, apple and fruit butters, honey, molasses, maple syrup, barley malt, organic eggs, goat's milk, soy milk, unsweetened fruit juices, vegetable juices, kefir, low-fat plain yogurt, protein powder, agar-agar (natural thickener), kuzu thickener, rice syrup, amasake sweetener, barley malt sweetener, roasted beans and grains.

Structuring Your Diet

	% of Daily Kilocalories (KCAL)	
Carbohydrates: complex (starches)	60–80%	
simple (sweets)	0–10%	= 100%
Protein (animal and vegetable)	10–20%	
Fats (animal and vegetable)	5–30%	

*28 grams = 1 ounce   16 ounces = 1 pound
3,500 calories (KCAL) = one pound of extra body weight!

Suggested Examples:

Carbohydrates (four KCAL per gram)—whole grains and cereals (brown rice, buckwheat, whole wheat, millet, oats, barley, wholegrain and vegetable pasta, egg-free noodles, bread, muffins, rolls, pancakes), fruit (one to three pieces daily), vegetables, potatoes, beans/legumes, one hundred percent fruit juice (limited four to six ounces daily—plus water)

Proteins (four KCAL per gram)—skim milk, low-fat (one percent or two percent), cheeses, milk and plain yogurts, eggs (use whites if you have a cholesterol problem), fresh fish, poultry (remove skin), veal, red meat on occasion (lean cuts only): lamb, beef, pork, venison

Essentials of Basic Healthful Eating

Fats (nine KCAL per gram; one tsp. = approx. five grams)—cold-pressed (natural) vegetable oils (safflower, sunflower, corn), olive oil (extra virgin is best), canola, sesame oil, edible grade flaxseed (linseed) oil, peanut oil, nuts, seeds, nutbutters (these also contain high protein), natural butter and "Better Butter." (Mix one half butter [softened at room temperature] with one half cold-pressed vegetable oil and refrigerate. Use "sparingly" in place of margarine [which is unhealthful] or regular butter.)

Sample Day:

Breakfast
- Hot or cold cereal (whole grain) with 1 tbsp. raisins or slivered almonds (oatmeal, Wheatena, oat, rice or wheat bran, millet, kasha)
- 1 piece of fresh fruit (or small glass of one hundred percent fruit juice)
- Hot decaf beverage

Lunch
- Tossed salad (on side: oil and vinegar)
- Rice-bean dish
- 1 piece fruit
- Natural beverage

Dinner
- Fresh fish (trout, flounder, sole, salmon)
- Baked potato with 1 pat "better butter" or 1 tbsp. non- or low-fat yogurt
- Steamed broccoli/carrots with lemon
- Natural beverage
- Tossed salad (on side: natural dressing)

Bulking Up with Fiber for Better Health

Fiber is an essential key to weight control and the avoidance and management of a broad array of health problems. Fiber can help us to lower cholesterol (especially guar-gum fibers), reduce constipation and lower our risk for various intestinal problems and cancers.

High-Fiber Foods

High-fiber and bran cereals
Beans/legumes
Broccoli
Cauliflower
Leafy green vegetables
Corn, oats and grains
Brown rice
Starchy vegetables
Wholewheat bread
Lightly cooked or fresh vegetables
Fresh or dried fruits
Nuts
Guar gum and pectin
Glucomannan

Fiber is especially helpful for diabetics, for weight control, for removing excess cholesterol and for preventing colorectal cancer.

Vitamins and Minerals

Vitamins and minerals are not only essential to our growth, vitality and well-being, but also to life itself. Although many people automatically equate these nutrients with supplemental pills and formulas, vitamins and minerals should first be obtained from our diet.

According to Dr. Daniel T. Quigley, author of *National Malnutrition* (1981), "Everyone who in the past has eaten sugar, white flour, or canned food, has some deficiency disease, depending on the percentage of such deficient food in the diet."

Reheating and overcooking foods at home or in res-

Essentials of Basic Healthful Eating

taurants can create nutrient losses of vitamins A, B, C and assorted minerals, including calcium. Even enriched products are deceptively promoted, since this process generally removes about twenty-two natural nutrients and replaces only three or four.

What's the answer? Selective food shopping, careful preparation and the addition of nutritional supplements as professionally suggested for your condition, or in a basic multivitamin-mineral as a form of health maintenance and insurance. Supplements are helpers for the body, not substitutes for food. Although many people think supplements can replace food, they cannot. In fact, vitamins and minerals require food for their proper assimilation in the body. Thus, function is analogous to an automobile's combustion, in which these key nutrients work like spark plugs, energizing and regulating our bodies as they work with the carbohydrates, fats and proteins we obtain in a properly structured and balanced unprocessed, whole-foods diet.

Taking food supplements in special combinations is often crucial to specially formulated health programs. Isolated supplements, used in orthomolecular medicine and psychiatry, are essential to balancing the metabolism when diet alone cannot be a sole dietary remedy. Increasing certain foods high in important nutrients is also vital to the success of a therapeutic nutritional plan.

Nutritional health depends on foods rich in vital nutrients. Here's a list of some foods that are powerhouse suppliers in the diet! How's your intake of these key components?

Vitamins

Vitamin A (Retinol or beta-carotene)—liver, fish oils, egg yolks, green and yellow vegetables, such as spinach, carrots, squash, yams, and yellow fruits, such as apricots

B vitamins B_1 (Thiamine)—whole grains, peas, Brazil nuts, sunflower seeds, soybeans, wheat germ

B_2 (Riboflavin)—liver, kelp, almonds, beet and turnip tops, leafy greens, milk, brewer's yeast

B_3 (Niacin)—whole grains, poultry, legumes, haddock, tuna, barley, peanuts, brewer's yeast

B_6 (Pyridoxine)—corn oil, brown rice, prunes, cabbage, whole grains, leafy greens, bananas, wheat bran, brewer's yeast.

B_{12} (Cyanocobalamin)—miso, tempeh, seafood, meat, kelp, dulse, dairy products

Folic acid—liver, nuts, spinach, lentils, turnip greens, beans, asparagus.

Pantothenic acid—whole grains, broccoli, legumes, salmon, liver, peanuts, brewer's yeast

Biotin: whole grains, lentils, eggs, liver, organ meats, banana, seafood, soy, peanuts, mushrooms, brewer's yeast.

Choline—whole grains, legumes, lecithin, soybeans, seafood

Inositol—grapefruit, oranges, fruit, vegetables, lecithin, nuts

PABA—wheat germ, rice bran, blackstrap molasses, eggs.

B_{15} (Pangamic acid or pangamate)—brown rice, sesame seeds, tahini, organ meats

Vitamin C (Ascorbic acid)—citrus fruits, broccoli, red and green peppers, turnip greens, cherries, parsley, cabbage, avocado, brussels sprouts

Vitamin D (Cholecalciferol)—salmon, cod liver oil, tuna, eggs, milk, butter and dairy products, wheat germ and even sunshine

Essentials of Basic Healthful Eating

Vitamin E (Tocopherol)—fish, meats, plant oils, nuts and seeds, peas, wheat germ oil, whole grains

Vitamin F (Unsaturated fatty acids)—butter; wheat germ; fish oils; cold-pressed vegetable, seed/nut and olive oils

Vitamin K (Phylloquinone)—eggs, cauliflower, seafood, soybeans, whole grains, greens and oats

Vitamin P (Bioflavonoids, Rutin, Hesperidin)—fruit, buckwheat, apricots, citrus

Minerals

Calcium—dark leafy greens, almonds, sesame, celery, kukicha twig tea, broccoli, soy, dairy

Phosphorus—seafood, squash, meats, whole grains, almonds, carrots, eggs, cheddar cheese

Magnesium—whole grains, tuna, pineapple, leafy greens, kelp, nuts, soybeans, molasses

Iron—lean meats, leafy green vegetables, raisins, figs, soybeans, eggs, liver, beans, oysters

Iodine—sea vegetables, beets, mushrooms, seafood, spinach, Irish moss, kelp, dulse, iodized salt

Potassium—oranges, bananas, leafy greens, tomatoes, whole grains, potato skins

Copper—raisins, legumes, organ meats, mushrooms, whole grains, seafood, cocoa

Manganese—bananas, leafy greens, celery, beets, pineapples, whole grains

Selenium—Garlic, onions, broccoli, whole grains, wheat germ, tuna, oysters, mushrooms, brewer's yeast, tomatoes, cabbage, bran

Chromium—corn oil, brewer's yeast, mushrooms, liver, beets, whole wheat, black pepper, apples, thyme

Cobalt—organ meats, oysters, clams, poultry, milk, green leafy vegetables, fruits

Chlorine—table salt, seafood, meats, ripe olives, rye flour

Fluoride—tea, seafood, fluoridated water, bone meal

Molybdenum—legumes, whole-grain cereals, milk, liver, dark green vegetables

Sulfur—fish, eggs, meats, cabbage, brussels sprouts

Vanadium—fish and seafood, vegetable oils, whole grains, liver

Zinc—beef, oatmeal, dark chicken, fish, beef liver, dried beans, bran, tuna, whole grains, mushrooms, nuts, pumpkin seeds, meats.

Amino Acids

The word "protein" is derived from the Greek word "proteios"—the most fundamental and important, or first.

Just a glance into a mirror will show you protein in the form of skin, hair, nails, teeth and even your eyes. Internally, too, your bones, arteries, organs, muscles and genes all carry protein. Although nutrients such as carbohydrates and fats are necessary to sustain life, only protein can build cells and repair tissue.

At the basis of protein's composition are amino acids (polypeptides), which combine to form chains, or long patterns, for other protein chains. Over one hundred amino acids occur in nature but only twenty-two are found in man, eight of which are considered "essential." Although all amino acids are necessary to health, the term "essential" means that these must be obtained from foods or supplements. If these eight are supplied at the same time, and in sufficient quantity, the other fourteen will be manufactured by the body.

Essentials of Basic Healthful Eating

Amino Acids

Essential

Isoleucine	Phenylalanine
Leucine	Threonine
Lysine	Tryptophan
Methionine	Valine

Nonessential

Alanine	Histidine*
Arginine*	Hydroxyglutamic acid
Aspartic acid	Hydroxyproline
Cysteine	Norleucine
Cystine	Proline
Glutamic acid	Serine
Glycine	Tyrosine

*May also be essential for infants and some individuals.

Besides building cells and repairing tissue, proteins also help to form antibodies to fight infections, viruses and bacteria. They also help the body to manufacture enzymes, hormones and the genetic blueprint (RNA and DNA) that accounts for our unique makeup. Protein also enhances the transport of oxygen throughout the body and supports muscular tone and function.

Although protein is obtained from various foods, such as fish, fowl, eggs, dairy products, meat, beans, nuts and seeds, and to some extent whole grains, we sometimes require particular amino acids to support us with special nutritional needs. The therapeutic effects of foods are limited by the brain barrier, which limits the amino acids that can enter the brain and the quantities permitted to enter. Because of this, no one amino acid can enter the brain after we ingest and then assimilate the food. The result is that the influence of any one or any particular combination of amino acids will have only a very slight or relatively no particularly therapeutic influence.

Because of this phenomenon, some health-care practitioners may choose to use a combination of dietary adjustments and the added benefit of particular amino acids for desired effects.

The use of these nutrients, as with most nutrients, should be closely regulated in accordance with an individual's health profile and whether or not he or she is taking particular drugs or medications. Although nutrients are food substances necessary to life and to our optimal functioning, they are uniquely different than drugs, and may potentially create unwelcome interactions if taken with some medications or with particular conditions.

For this reason, appropriate supervision is always suggested prior to using isolated amino acids or other nutrients in therapeutic amounts.

Common Food Sources of the Essential Amino Acids

Isoleucine—Beef, chicken, fish, soybeans, soy protein, ham, pork, vegetable patty, eggs, cottage cheese, liver, baked beans, milk

Leucine—Beef, chicken, soy protein, fish, soybeans, ham, pork, cottage cheese, liver, vegetable patty, eggs, baked beans

Lysine—Chicken, beef, fish, ham, pork, soy protein, soybeans, cottage cheese, baked beans, eggs, goat's

Essentials of Basic Healthful Eating

milk, milk, peanuts, vegetable patty, yeast (brewer's), oatmeal

Methionine—Chicken, beef, fish, ham, pork, eggs, cottage cheese, liver, soybeans, soy protein, vegetable patty, sardines, milk, yogurt

Phenylalanine—Soy protein, beef, chicken, soybeans, fish, vegetable patty, eggs, cottage cheese, baked beans, peanuts, almonds, milk

Threonine—Beef, chicken, fish, ham, pork, soy protein, soybeans, liver, eggs, cottage cheese, goat's milk, baked beans, vegetable patty

Tryptophan—Beef, soy protein, chicken, soybeans, fish, eggs, vegetable patty, cottage cheese, milk, mixed nuts, baked beans

Valine—Beef, chicken, fish, soy protein, soybeans, ham, pork, eggs, liver, vegetable patty, cottage cheese, baked beans, milk.

Supplements and Drugs: Some Don't Mix

The use of certain medications or supplements may be very necessary for your health, yet certain precautions are often necessary. A recent FDA survey found about forty percent of adults routinely take supplements and many of these people need to know that many drugs can destroy the vitamins or interact with them in a harmful way.

NUTRITION AS BASIS OF GOOD HEALTH

Drugs and Vitamins That Don't Mix*

Nutritional Supplement	When Taken With	May Possibly Cause	Additional Remarks
Vitamin A (Carotene)	*Accutane*, used for acne	Headache, nausea and visual problems	ACCUTANE is a vitamin A derivative; additive toxicity
Vitamin B6 (Pyridoxine)	*Larodopa* (levodopa), used for Parkinsonism	Decreased benefit from medication	Well established; no problem with SINEMET
	Phenobarbital or Dilantin (phenytoin), for	Reduced seizure control	Observed in patients taking more than 200 mg. of B6 per day
Vitamin C (Ascorbic acid)	*Coumadin* (warfarin), a blood-thinning drug	Increased risk of blood clotting	Believed to be due to diarrhea from high doses of vitamin C
	Estinyl (estrogen) or birth control pills	Increased sex hormone side effect	Breakthrough bleeding may occur after stopping vitamin C
	Prolixin a phenothiazine-type tranquilizer	Mental state worsened	Occurred with only a one-gram dose of vitamin C
Vitamin D (Calciferol)	*Calan, Isoptin* (verapamil), used for angina and chest pain	Decreased heart effect	Only when also combined with high doses of calcium
Vitamin E (Alpha-tocopherol)	Prescription prenatal vitamins with iron	Decreased iron supplement benefit	Vitamin E reduces the iron uptake
	Coumadin (warfarin), a blood-thinning drug	Increased bleeding tendency	Can be serious! A lower Coumadin dose may be necessary.

*1986 Patient Medication Bulletin, P.O. Box 14281, Torrance, CA 90503.

Essentials of Basic Healthful Eating

Tyramine-rich Foods—
Dietary Restriction for Migraine
and MAO Patients

ALERT: These foods, nutrients and medications must be avoided if you are taking MAO (Monoamine oxidase inhibitor) drugs. An interaction between this type of drug and foods and beverages rich in tyramine could cause serious hypertensive crisis, nosebleeds and potentially lethal strokes or heart attacks. Tyramine is an amino acid made in the body from tyrosine. Other nutrients (special) or medications listed could also be dangerous.

MAO Drug Names—Actomol, Catron, Drazine, Eutonyl, Furozone, Marplan, Marsilid, Nardil, Miamid, Parnate and Tersavid (or as listed and prescribed)

Generic MAO Names—Furazolidone, iproniazid, isocarboxazid, mebanazine, nialamide, pargyline, phenelzine, pheniprazine, phenoxypropazine, piohydrazine and tranylcypromine (or as listed and prescribed)

Avoid the following foods and beverages, which are rich in tyramine. The other substances on the list are also of possible danger to individuals taking MAO medications.

Fruits—Avocados, apples, raisins, bananas, canned figs, strawberries, raspberries

Meats, Fowl and Fish—Meat products (sausage, pepperoni), regular and aged pork, beef, bacon, fish (especially various aged types), canned fish, chicken and poultry, liver and liverwurst (chicken, liver and pork), eggs, anchovies, pickled herring, dried and salted fish, caviar, snails, cured beef, salami (Any high-protein aged food may also present a hazard.)

Bakery Products

Beverages—Beer, wine, cola, cocoa, vermouth, cognac, coffee

Dairy Products—Milk, sour cream, whey, yogurt, butter and cheese (Generally, cottage cheese, cream cheese and some plain yogurt are safe to eat.)

Other Foods—Soy sauce, mushrooms, yeast extract, broad beans and pods, chocolate, meat tenderizers, "Bovril" extract, "Marmite" extract, some grains, various "Italian dishes," dishes and dressing with cheese, beets, sauerkraut, Worcestershire sauce, licorice, junket, curry powder, some salad dressings (especially Italian)

Nutrients—Tyrosine, phenylalanine, tryptophan

Other Drugs and Medications—Cold medications, nasal/sinus decongestants, asthma inhalants, diet (anti-appetite) medicine, levadopa, dopamine, local anesthetics with epinephrine (direct and indirect and combination types), sympathomimetic amines (check with M.D.), tyramine.

ALWAYS ASK YOUR PHYSICIAN FOR ADDITIONAL ADVICE AND SPECIFIC GUIDELINES.

Part Two:
BALANCING YOUR LIFESTYLE WITH EXERCISE AND LIVING

WELLNESS THROUGH MORE BALANCED LIVING

Your body is your thought in a form you can see.
—RICHARD BACH,
Jonathan Livingston Seagull

EATING WELL is a vital component to health enhancement, but to more fully assess the dynamics of good health, we also need to be in touch with our total self. This means becoming aware of the role that rest, physical exercise, stress management and emotional and spiritual balance all play in our health.

Getting sufficient exercise is a major key to assisting our bodies' use of the nutrients we are feeding them. Exercise (especially aerobic forms) lowers cholesterol, improves cardiovascular tone, promotes weight loss and reduces day-to-day stress. It also helps us nutritionally by assisting nutrient delivery by improved circulation throughout the body. Most exercise authorities generally agree that exercise should be included in our daily routine with stretching, walking and similar forms of limbering movements. More strenuous exercise should, however, with medical approval, be included at least three to five times weekly for at least fifteen minutes to an hour per session. This form should be vigorous enough to increase aerobic heart rates to sixty to ninety percent of maximum training heart rate levels.

This can be easily determined by following a special heart-rate formula based on pulse rate taken before, during and after exercise.

Maximum and Training Heart Rates by Age

Age	Maximum Heart Rate	Training Zone 60% Rate	80% Rate	90% Rate
20	200	120	160	180
25	195	117	156	175
30	190	114	152	171
35	185	111	148	166
40	180	108	144	162
45	175	105	140	157
50	170	102	136	153
55	165	99	132	149
60	160	96	128	144
65	155	93	124	140

How to Find Your Training Heart Rate

For exercise to be aerobic, it must be performed at *your training heart rate for twenty to sixty minutes, three to five days per week.* The American College of Sports Medicine recommends that you use this heart rate to determine the intensity of your workouts. Since this rate differs from person to person, use the following formula to find your personal training rate.

Wellness Through Balanced Living

Training Heart Rate

    220
- ____ minus your age
- = maximum heart rate
- − ____ minus your resting heart rate
  (See the next section for instructions on determining resting heart rate.)
- = maximum heart rate reserve
- × 0.7 multiply by 0.7 (used to determine 70 percent of your maximum heart rate reserve)
- + ____ plus your resting heart rate
- = your training heart rate

Sample Training Heart Rate

Profile: A thirty-year-old woman whose resting heart rate is seventy beats per minute:

    220
− 30 her age
  190 her maximum heart rate
− 70 her resting heart rate
  120 her maximum heart rate reserve
× 0.7
  84.0
+ 70 her resting heart rate
  154 her training heart rate

Your Resting Heart Rate

Resting heart rate can be a good indicator of the health of your cardiovascular system and your fitness level. Locate your carotid artery with the tips of your fingers—it's in the front strip of muscle running vertically down your neck—or find your radial artery by pressing your fingers on the inside of your wrist just below your wrist bone. Take your pulse for one minute.

    Very fit ....Under 50
    Fit 50–70
    Average 70–80
    Unfit ....80 and up

How to Take Your Exercise Pulse Rate

1. Take your exercise pulse rate *immediately* after exercising by counting the number of times your heart beats in 10 seconds.
2. Then multiply your pulse by 6. For example, if your heart beats 30 times in 10 seconds, multiply 30 by 6; your exercise pulse rate would be 180.

Take your pulse every five or ten minutes during aerobic exercise. If it's high, then slow down. If low, speed up a little to get training benefits.

Exercise—Some Varied Forms

Aerobic
1. Demands large amounts of oxygen for prolonged periods of time at steady rate, generally rhythm in breathing is created
2. Positive training results: marathoners can raise basal metabolic rate (BMR) twelve to fifteen times resting rate, thus increasing blood volume and improving oxygen transport, lung capacity and endurance, heart muscle strength and blood pumping capacity; increases in HDL, "Good Cholesterol"

Wellness Through Balanced Living

3. Examples: jogging, running, speed walking, aerobic dancing, cross-country skiing, swimming, cycling
4. Excellent cardiovascular conditioning and strengthening, life extension and weight control benefits

Anaerobic
1. Meaning "without oxygen," this form of exercise is performed without utilizing the oxygen you are breathing
2. "Threshold" defines difference between this and aerobic forms
3. Examples: a 100-yard dash—totally anaerobic
   sprinting for first 2–3 minutes to exhaustion
4. Good speed, increase development

Isometric
1. Joints and muscles don't move
2. Muscles don't contract—they stay the same length
3. Examples: pushing, pulling, lifting
4. Can build muscle size and strength—but *caution* for increases in blood pressure, heart attack and cardiac irregularity

Isotonic or Isophasic (Dynamic)
1. Joint or extremity movement
2. Muscles do contract
3. Examples: weight lifting and calisthenics (*i.e.*, Nautilus)
4. Can build muscle mass and strength, but do little for the cardiovascular system. They *fail* to build long-distance endurance, increase blood volume and lung capacity or lower pulse or blood pressure

Isokinetic
1. Weight lifting through an entire range of motion and return to position—emphasis on rehabilitation (accommodates muscle output, less resistance to force)
2. Unlike isotonic, gravity plays no prominent part

3. Examples: Circuit weight training (generally consisting of ten stations with twelve to fifteen repetitions with a thirty-second period); two sets of ten exercises in twenty minutes four times a week is a typical schedule (*i.e.*, Cybex)
4. Can build muscle, strength and power (emphasis on constant velocity, constant single speed)

Exercise is also a key component to weight control. Combined with a low-fat, high–complex carbohydrate diet you can greatly offset your risks for many weight-related health problems.

The following charts illustrate your caloric burn rates in various forms of exercise. You can also see where you stand in terms of body weight and health risks.

Estimated Calories Per Hour Used During Certain Activities

Type of Activity	*Calories Used Per Hour*	*Examples*
Sedentary	10–40	Reading, watching TV, writing, eating, sewing, playing cards, miscellaneous office work
Light	50–100	Office and other activities requiring some standing and arm movement, preparing and cooking food, dusting, hand-washing clothes, ironing
Moderate	110–180	Light housework (making beds, mopping, scrubbing, sweeping, light polishing and waxing), light gardening and carpenty work, walking moderately fast

Wellness Through Balanced Living

Vigorous	190–270	Heavy housework (heavy scrubbing and waxing, hanging laundry, stripping beds), walking fast, bowling, golfing, dancing, riding, skating, doing calisthenics
Strenuous	300–700+	Heavy manual labor, cycling fast, swimming, climbing, jogging, running, playing tennis, skiing

Adapted from *Patient Care*, May 1, 1973.

National Institute of Aging
1985 Weight Recommendations for Both Sexes
(in pounds by age in years)

Height	**20–29**	**30–39**	**40–49**	**50–59**	**60–69**
4'10"	84–111	92–119	99–127	107–135	115–142
4'11"	87–115	95–123	103–131	111–139	119–147
5'	90–119	98–127	106–135	114–143	123–152
5'1"	93–123	101–131	110–140	118–148	127–157
5'2"	96–127	105–136	113–144	122–153	131–163
5'3"	99–131	108–140	117–149	126–158	135–165
5'4"	102–135	112–145	121–154	130–163	140–173
5'5"	106–140	115–149	125–159	134–168	144–179
5'6"	109–144	119–154	129–164	138–174	148–184
5'7"	112–148	122–159	133–169	143–179	153–190
5'8"	116–153	126–163	137–174	147–184	158–196
5'9"	119–157	130–168	141–179	151–190	162–201
5'10"	122–162	134–173	145–184	156–195	167–207
5'11"	126–167	137–178	149–190	160–201	172–213
6'	129–171	141–183	153–195	165–207	177–219
6'1"	133–176	145–188	157–200	169–213	182–225
6'2"	137–181	149–194	162–206	174–219	187–232
6'3"	141–186	153–199	166–212	179–225	192–238
6'4"	144–191	157–205	171–218	184–231	197–244

Source: Gerontology Research Center for National Institute of Aging, 1986.

How to Measure Your Body

The following measurement sites are good indicators for weight loss or gain:

>Women (aged 17–35): abdomen, right thigh, right forearm
>Women (aged 36 and up): abdomen, right thigh, calf
>Men (aged 17–35): right upper arm, abdomen, right forearm
>Men (aged 36 and up): buttocks, abdomen, right forearm

In measuring, follow these guidelines:

>Abdomen: ½ inch above the navel
>Buttocks: maximum protrusion with heels together
>Right thigh: upper thigh just below the buttocks
>Right upper arm: arm straight, palm out and extended in front of the body (measure midway between the shoulder and the elbow)
>Right forearm: widest circumference between the elbow and the wrist
>Right calf: widest circumference midway between the ankle and the knee

Your measurements (three sites, taken every seven days):

Date:_____	Date:_____	Date:_____
1)_____	1)_____	1)_____
2)_____	2)_____	2)_____
3)_____	3)_____	3)_____

Wellness Through Balanced Living

Is Your Weight Hindering Your Health?

(Increase in Risk)

	20 to 30% Overweight	*40% or More Overweight*	*Deaths Per Year*
Cancer			
Male			
Colon/Rectum	26%	73%	29,100
Prostate	37%	29%	26,100
Female			
Breast	16%	53%	39,900
Cervix	51%	139%	6,800
Endometrium	85%	442%	2,900
Gallbladder	74%	258%	5,300
Ovary	9%	63%	11,600
Diabetes			
Male	156%	419%	14,859*
Female	234%	690%	21,928*
Heart Disease			
Male	32%	95%	289,461
Female	39%	107%	251,857
Stroke			
Male	17%	127%	61,697
Female	16%	52%	92,630

Sources: *J. Chron. Dis.* 32:563, 1979; *Personal Communication*, John Lubers, American Cancer Society; Kathy Santini, National Center for Health Statistics.

*This figure does not include the many diabetics who die of heart disease.

Good Diet Structure for Weight Control and Optimum Health

		Calorie Breakdown		
		10–20% Protein	*60% Carbohydrate*	*10–30% Fat*
800	Calories (very low, semistarvation for very limited time)	80–160	480	80–240
1,000		100–200	600	100–300
1,200	(lowest suggested level for maintenance or loss)	120–240	720	120–360
1,500		150–300	900	150–450
1,800		180–360	1080	180–360
2,000		200–400	1200	200–600
2,500		250–500	1500	250–750
3,000		300–600	1800	300–900

GETTING IN TOUCH WITH THE INNER SELF

Only he who knows the innermost nature of man can cure him in earnest.
—PARACELSUS

ONE REASON why exercise helps us to energize, unwind and relieve stress is that we diminish excess adrenalin. According to research, the role of stress on our health can be devastating, creating a link or basis for a diverse array of illnesses.

Stress is commonly defined as intense exertion, strain or effort. Basically, it is the wear and tear of life. In fact, without stress, life could not exist. The birth of a child, the first day of school, a work deadline, a traffic jam, a vacation, a body fighting to regain health are all examples of stress. Stress can be perceived as the spice of life or, depending upon circumstances and an individuals' capacities and reactions, it can have damaging side effects that may lead to premature aging, disease, accidents and, sometimes, to a shortened life. Stress can be mental, emotional or physical, all having some impact—sometimes good, sometimes harmful.

Today, it is estimated that over seventy-five percent of all visits to physicians have stress as a major underlying component. This tells us that most people in today's society face emotional problems in coping with the events of their lives. In fact, one out of six Americans takes some form of antianxiety sedative regularly, with Valium and Librium being the two most widely prescribed drugs in the United States.

Life Stressors

Researchers Holmes and Rahe (1967) published a scale of social readjustment that profiled the impact of various life events upon individuals. Depending upon the total value of events experienced over a period of twelve months, the risk for illness, destructive behavioral patterns or other stress-connected responses could be determined.

Social Readjustment Scale

Life Event	Mean Value
1. Death of spouse	100
2. Divorce	73
3. Marital separation	65
4. Jail term	63
5. Death of close family member	63
6. Personal injury or illness	53
7. Marriage	50
8. Fired at work	47
9. Marital reconciliation	45
10. Retirement	45
11. Change in health of family member	44
12. Pregnancy	40
13. Sex difficulties	39
14. Gain of new family member	39
15. Business readjustment	39

Getting in Touch with Inner Self

16.	Change in financial state	39
17.	Death of close friend	37
18.	Change to different line of work	36
19.	Change in number of arguments with spouse	35
20.	Mortgage over $10,000 (adjust to current equivalent)	31
21.	Foreclosure of mortgage or loan	30
22.	Change in responsibilities at work	29
23.	Son or daughter leaving home	29
24.	Trouble with in-laws	29
25.	Outstanding personal achievement	28
26.	Wife begins or stops work	26
27.	Begin or end of school	26
28.	Change in living conditions	25
29.	Revision of personal habits	24
30.	Trouble with boss	23
31.	Change in work hours or conditions	20
32.	Change in residence	20
33.	Change in schools	20
34.	Change in recreation	19
35.	Change in religious activities	19
36.	Change in social activities	18
37.	Mortgage or loan less than $10,000 (adjust to current equivalent)	17
38.	Change in sleeping habits	16
39.	Change in number of family get-togethers	15
40.	Change in eating habits	15
41.	Vacation	13
42.	Christmas	12
43.	Minor violations of the law	11

Total Value of Events Experienced Over Twelve Months:

Approximately		*Possible Implications*
150–300	50%	50% risk stress-response over following twenty-four months
300+	80%	80% risk stress-response over following twenty-four months

Source: Holmes, T. H. and Rahe, R. H.: The Social readjustment rating scale. *J. Psychosom. Res. 11*:213–218, 1967.

Emotional and physical stress are basic to our life experiences. An awareness of the type of stress that will provide us with health and pleasurable exhilaration, homeostasis or disease needs to be understood.

Stressors
(Typical Examples)

A. *Eustress* (healthy, good stress)
- moderate exercise
- love
- happiness
- fulfillment (personal or professional)

B. *Neustress* (homeostatic, neutral stress)
- walking
- talking
- breathing

C. *Distress* (disease-provoking, bad stress)
- overexertion
- injury
- disease/illness
- surgery
- death of a loved one
- divorce or separation
- loss of job
- financial problems
- frustration
- anxiety
- boredom or helplessness/hopelessness

As we see, harmful stress is almost like an attack upon our physical or emotional centers. Sudden events and strong emotions set off an alarm reaction from the nervous system. This process originates deep in the brain centers. It is from here that the pituitary alerts the body with ACTH, a hormone that regulates

Getting in Touch with Inner Self

the emergency mechanisms of the adrenal glands situated just above the kidneys. These glands, in turn, send out hormones (corticosteroids), which prepare the body to handle the emergency. When we continually manifest persistent stress, intensity or negative emotions (such as fear, anger, frustration or impatience), we can produce excessive amounts of adrenalin and toxic body chemicals that greatly reduce the long-term overall strength and resilience of our bodies. As a result, we may experience a variety of symptoms as a signal to warn us that a destructive process is occurring. When we fail to take heed of such warnings, we can ultimately set ourselves up for illness or disease.

One aspect of such studies seems evident; that is, the happier we are with ourselves and our life, the

10 Warning Signs of Mental Illness
(National Alliance for the Mentally Ill)

1. Confused thinking
2. Persistent depression
3. Excessive worry, anxiety or fear
4. Unexpected change in personality or mood
5. Withdrawal from others
6. Thinking or talking of suicide
7. Violent thoughts or behavior
8. Changes in eating or sleeping patterns
9. Increased use of alcohol or drugs
10. Difficulty coping with daily activities, school, job or personal needs.

At any given time, 1 in 5 Americans (estimated number) has mental disturbance enough to require psychiatric care. (Ed Edelson, December 30, 1985, *New York Post*)

greater our mental health. Most simply, we may see that HAPPINESS = MENTAL HEALTH!

Health and medical practitioners increasingly recognize the importance of emotions in influencing health. The mind and body work together interdependently— *not* as separate units. Studies continually illustrate the relationship of the mind upon the body, and the body upon the mind. This awareness is the basis of psychosomatic medicine. (Mind ["psyche"] + body ["soma"] = psychosomatic.)

Many people think that a psychosomatic illness is just a harmless condition that will not create physical damage. This notion is false. Emotions cause changes in the body, from subtle blushing to the pounding of our heart. Hidden (subconscious) feelings, deep-seated emotional conflicts, problems too difficult to face and prolonged emotional tensions all influence our health.

Physicians commonly find that emotions experienced by patients are significantly linked to a broad array of ailments, either as a causal agent or as a factor worsening the condition.

Common Stress Indicators and Potential Linked Conditions

1. Maladjustment to life-change events (personal, social or professional)
2. Fatigue or sleeping difficulties
3. Irritability, impatience, aggressive or competitive behavior
4. Emotional difficulties
5. Headaches
6. Nervousness or emotionally rooted habits or responses (*e.g.*, smoking, substance abuse, tics)

Getting in Touch with Inner Self

7. Social or behavioral change (*e.g.*, withdrawal or overinvolvement, maladaptive or antisocial behavior)
8. Joint or muscle pain, weakness, or stiffness
9. Obsessive and/or compulsive behavior, rigidity, etc.
10. Breathing difficulties
11. Changes in physical appearance, personal hygiene, self-image or self-esteem
12. Changes in heart rate, rhythm, or blood pressure
13. Increased, recurrent or chronic problems (allergies, colds, accidents, sexual problems, etc.)
14. Physical or emotional trauma
15. Inability to relax, do nothing, or "let go" without feeling guilty
16. Hormonal imbalances
17. Circulatory problems
18. Digestive problems (ulcers, colitis, constipation)
19. Impaired immunity
20. Menstrual-related tension, pain or irregularities.

Coping with life, our emotions, fears and conflicts takes courage and insight. Often we are unable to break through the destructive habits and response patterns we have established without professional assistance. Just as we get checkups and advice on improving our physical health, so, too, should we regularly address our mental health and the thoughts, emotions, conflicts, habits and behaviors that may be key factors in our physical ailments and obstacles to our personal growth. We often need to recognize the value in learning new skills and ways to improve our life and our well-being, rather than falsely depending on a pill or tranquilizer to mask an ongoing problem. Depending on such symptom blockers, without addressing the real problems we have, can be likened to removing the oil light in our car when it continually flashes. We may not see the warning light any longer, but we are still burning out the engine.

To understand stress management, it is helpful to first assess how we transform a stressful situation into a stress reaction. The sequence of stress can be illustrated as follows:

Stressor	**Perception**	**Stress**
Event	Your thoughts	How you feel
Situation	Your evaluation	How you react
Pressure	Your beliefs	
Demand	Your interpretation	
Example:		
Extra assignment at work	"This is overwhelming." "I can't stand this."	Anger
		Annoyance
		Body tenses
		Depressed
		Headache
		Hyperventilation (lightheaded effect)
		Moodiness
		Stomach or intestinal distress
		Upset

In this example, we see that perception is a key to controlling the situation. In other words, your perception governs how your body responds, and it is here, with your way of thinking or mentally reacting, that can determine if the stress will ultimately harm you.

Although counseling or psychotherapy are often vital to the success of stress management for many

Getting in Touch with Inner Self

people, for many others simply understanding the significance of a stressor or situation and understanding our response intensity and how to lessen it is often a major step. For example, in this situation was the extra assignment worth the type of response it was given? On a scale of 1 to 10, perhaps it was worth 4 and we gave it a 10 response. Certainly we would then have "overreacted." Perhaps if we viewed the situation as a positive challenge, it would have been perceived differently and been rated more accordingly.

Characteristic Behaviors

Type A
- Rapid movements and speech
- Impatience
- Domineering and competitive
- Obsessive-compulsive behavior
- Guilty feeling if relaxing
- Overconcern with getting things done
- Little concern/time with developing inner qualities
- Nervous gestures
- Inner hostility and anger
- Controlling behavior and rigidity in thought and functioning

Type B
- No Type A characteristics
- No time urgency or obsessiveness
- Enjoy fun and relaxation without guilt
- No hostility
- "Roll with punches" attitude
- Content with self
- Seeks meaningful associations
- Easy-going personality

BALANCING YOUR LIFESTYLE

This reminds us of how our thinking errors often help create undue stress. Such reactions also tie into personality. Generally, personality types illustrate categories of individuals who show characteristics of high-stress profiles. Personality types are good pictures of the basic makeup of people, yet these makeups and problems can change with awareness and effort.

In general, many people equate the Type A with the hard-driving heart attack personality, and Type B with the calmer and generally healthier (physically and mentally) individual. Although many people display characteristics of both the A and B types, most people in our society seem to be more like Type A, thus synonymous with stressful makeups. Studies also indicate that personality may be strongly linked to various health conditions, such as allergies, arthritis, arrythmias and other conditions. Other works also suggest that a Type C—cancer-prone personality—may also exist.

Ways to Help Yourself De-Stress

- Take a leisurely stroll
- Enjoy nature (sailing, hiking, biking, camping)
- Find an enjoyable hobby (art, music, cooking, photography)
- Talk-it-out with a friend
- Take time to appreciate what really matters in life
- Get in touch with the inner you—self-awareness
- Take steps to improve the neglected parts of your life
- Build closer ties with family and friends
- Begin a regular exercise program
- Improve your diet and living patterns
- Pamper yourself—try a massage, facial or sauna
- Form a support group to discuss important topics
- Take a personal growth-enhancing course

Getting in Touch with Inner Self

- Get away for a weekend or a vacation
- Give and receive comforting hugs!

Professional Assistance to Help You De-Stress

- Biofeedback therapy
- Relaxation exercises (breathing, meditation, imagery-visualization)
- Stress management education
- Individual or group counseling
- Psychotherapy

Learning to relax is often critical to Type A and, in general, to most stressful people. Assessing the way we think, act and feel is the basis to stress management. Making positive growth-enhancing steps and goals for our health and life is also important. Learning to relax is yet another.

Relaxation training is the basis to biofeedback training, a process by which individuals see and hear how their stress and tension responses are affecting their body. A basic exercise to beginning biofeedback training is diaphragmatic breathing. This method of improved breathing concentrates on utilizing the entire lung cavity to supply your body with the fullest nourishment of oxygen and the more complete exhange of oxygen and carbon dioxide. Unlike stressful breathing (often called emergency breathing), which uses only the upper portions of the lung, the complete breath helps you to automatically relax.

Now, observe your breathing. How deep is it? How slow and steady is each inhalation and exhalation?

Read the following exercise carefully and practice this twice daily or whenever you are anxious or feeling highly stressful.

BALANCING YOUR LIFESTYLE

Directions for the Complete Breath

Benefits: provides quick anxiety relief, increases vitality, soothes nerves, strengthens intestinal and abdominal muscles, relieves asthma, emphysema, shortness of breath. It is often not recommended for people who have peptic ulcer, hernia or hyperthyroid.

Step 1: Sit in a relaxed position, or practice by lying flat on your back with your knees up, feet flat on the floor or bed, slightly apart.
Step 2: Place your hands lightly on your abdomen.
Step 3: Breathe in through your nose and expand only your abdomen. Watch your fingertips part.
Step 4: Exhale and contract your abdomen. Feel your fingertips meet.
Step 5: Practice this abdominal breath ten times. Do not strain. Let your breath flow in and out with ease. Listen to your breath go in and out. Visualize yourself relaxing as you exhale.
Step 6: Place your hands on your rib cage.
Step 7: Inhale very slowly, watching your fingertips part.
Step 8: Very slowly exhale, contracting your rib cage.
Step 9: Practice this diaphragm breath ten times, very slowly.
Step 10: Place your fingertips on your collarbones.
Step 11: Raise your shoulders and inhale in the upper part of your chest. Feel your fingertips part.
Step 12: Exhale slowly and then practice the upper breath ten times.
Step 13: Place your hands, palms up, alongside your body.
Step 14: Put the three breaths together. Inhale slowly, expanding first the abdomen, then the diaphragm, then the upper chest. Hold.

Adapted From: *Enhancing Wellness*, by C. C. Clark, Spring Publishing, N.Y., 1981.

Getting in Touch with Inner Self

Step 15: Exhale, contracting first the abdomen, then the rib cage, then the upper chest.

Step 16: Repeat the Complete Breath until you establish a comfortable, relaxing rhythm. Concentrate on what is happening in your body as you breathe. Feel the old, bad air leave your body. Feel the clean, fresh air healing your body as you breathe in. Notice how relaxed and calm you are becoming.

When you have mastered the complete breath, continue to practice it twice daily without the use of your hands and integrate relaxing visualizations (a beach scene, mountain stream, or other pleasant image or experience) in your mind's eye.

Mastering breathing is step one in learning to relax within an in-depth relaxation or biofeedback program. As you perfect your breathing, integrate alternate relaxing thoughts and phrases and visualize yourself achieving the objectives of these phrases as you center and balance yourself more fully.

Breathing Phrases

> When the mind is disturbed, the multiplicity of things is produced, but when the mind is quieted, the multiplicity of things disappear.
> —ASHVAGHUSHA, *Awakening of Faith*

On Inhaling Breath	**On Relaxing Breath**
"I close my eyes	. . . and bring my thoughts inside."
"My breathing gets deeper	. . . and I quiet my thoughts."
"My body becomes still	. . . as my muscles relax."

BALANCING YOUR LIFESTYLE

"I focus on my inner self ... and release my tensions (fears, frustrations, anxieties)."

"I breathe in health ... and release disease (pain, infection, fatigue, discomfort, imbalance)."

Such exercises help to quiet the mind and sooth tension, thus removing much of our psychosomatic distress.

Living healthfully is a process of self-enrichment that allows you to enjoy a fuller life with more positive habits, thoughts and goals. Letting go of illness, including some of the benefits often derived from health problems (*i.e.*, extra attention, avoidance of situations and obligations) takes desire and courage; yet without this will and determination to be transformed, our health and total personal wellness can remain elusive.

> "A journey of three thousand miles is begun by a single step."—LAO-TZU.

That first step to better health is up to you. Welcome to a healthier life.

GLOSSARY OF COMMON HEALTH TERMS

Abdomen—Part of the body located between the diaphragm and the pelvis. Contains abdominal organs (viscera).

Acetone—Organic substance found in abnormal amounts in urine of diabetics. Acetone bodies are also called ketone bodies.

Acetylcholine—A chemical transmitter for nerve impulses that is released upon stimulation of the nerve and in the presence of calcium.

Adipose—Fat or containing fat, as in adipose tissue.

Adrenal—Endocrine gland located near the kidney, also called suprarenal.

Aerobic—Occurring in the presence of oxygen. An aerobic activity requires adequate oxygen to meet tissue demands.

Aldosterone—A steroid hormone produced by the adrenal cortex responsible for electrolyte (sodium-potassium) balance.

Allergy—Sensitivity to a substance (allergen) causing a variety of symptoms, such as bronchial asthma, sinus congestion or dermatitis.

Alveolar—Referring to jaw area or air cells of the lungs.

Amenorrhea—Absence or abnormal discontinuation of the menses.

Amino Acid—Building blocks of protein.

Amylase—Pancreatic or salivary enzyme that breaks down starch.

Anemia—Condition characterized as a deficiency of hemoglobin in red blood cells.

Anorexia—Lack, decline or loss of appetite. An eating disorder.

Antigen—Foreign substance, usually a protein, that produces an immune response.

Antioxidant—Substance that prevents or impedes oxidation.

Arrhythmia—Irregular heart beat.

Arteriosclerosis—"Hardening of the arteries." A variety of conditions that cause artery walls to thicken and lose elasticity.

Ataxia—Irregular muscle action.

Atherosclerosis—A form of arteriosclerosis. A depositing of fatty plaques along inner intimic artery wall, narrowing the channel and reducing blood supply.

ATP (Adenosine Triphosphate)—Energy current of the body.

Axilla—The armpit; hollow beneath the arm.

Basal Metabolic Rate—Energy required for cells to work when the body is at rest.

Bile—Fluid produced in the liver and stored in the gallbladder, that is secreted into intestines to emulsify fats during digestion.

Biofeedback—Various methods to feed back information regarding various physiological changes.

Biopsy—Removal of body tissue for microscopic study.

Bradycardia—Reduced beating of heart below 60 beats per minute in adults or below 120 in the fetus.

Bronchiole—Small division of lung tubes.

Bruxism—The destructive clenching and grinding of teeth with muscular tension.

Bulimia—Eating disorder characterized by gorging and purging.

Calorie—Unit of heat required to raise temperature of one gram of water to one degree centigrade.

Glossary

Capillaries—Small blood vessels containing the smallest arteries and veins.
Carbohydrate—A starch, sugar, cellulose or gum.
Carcinogen—A cancer-causing substance.
Cardiovascular Disease—Combination of heart and blood vessel disorders that include heart attack, stroke, atherosclerosis and congestive heart failure.
Carotid—Principal artery extending through neck and head.
Celiac—Relating or located in the abdomen.
Cerebellum—Part of the hindbrain that lies below the occipital part of the cerebrum on each side. Concerned with voluntary muscle movement.
Cerebrum—Largest part of the brain in upper part of cranium and having two hemispheres that are divided into lobes.
Cervix—Any neck or constricted part of an organ.
Cholesterol—A fatty substance or sterol found in all animal fats, bile, skin, blood and brain tissue.
Chyme—A mixture of partially digested food and stomach secretions.
Collagen—Protein substance that forms connective tissue and organic matrix in bones and teeth.
Coronary Occlusion—Obstruction or narrowing of one or more of the coronary arteries, hindering blood flow to receiving tissue.
Dehydration—Condition of excessive water loss from the body.
Diastole—Relaxing dilation period of the heart muscle.
Diverticulosis—Development of tiny sacs in weakened areas of the intestines.
Duodenum—Upper portion of small intestines.
Dyspnea—Difficult or labored breathing.
Eclampsia—Convulsions during pregnancy usually associated with edema, hypertension or proteinoria.
Edema—Presence of abnormal quantities of fluid in intercellular tissue spaces of body.
Elastin—Yellowish elastic protein in connective tissue.

Electrocardiograph—Instrument used for making records of heart's electric currents.

Electrolyte—Ionized form of an ion. Common electrolytes include sodium, potassium and chloride.

Embolism—Spontaneous blocking of an artery by a clot or free-floating obstruction.

Endocrine—Secreting to the inside, into either tissue fluid or blood.

Enriched—Description of processed food that has four nutrients (thiamin, riboflavin, niacin and iron) added back to replace those lost in refining.

Enzyme—Biological catalyst that initiates and accelerates chemical reactions.

Epithelium—A tissue that forms the outer part (epidermis) of the skin.

Erythrocyte—A mature red blood cell.

Essential Amino Acid—An amino acid that cannot be synthesized by the body and must be supplied by the diet.

Essential Fatty Acid—A fatty acid, such as linoleic acid, that cannot be made by the body and hence must be supplied regularly from the diet.

Eustachian Tube—Tube connecting inner ear with throat that helps equalize air pressure.

Exocrine—Secreting toward the outside, or away from, the secreting tissue by tubes or ducts.

Fallopian Tubes—Ducts connected to uterus. They carry ova from the ovaries to the uterine cavity and provide a place for reproductive fertilization.

Feces—Waste material discharged from bowel.

Fetus—The developing unborn baby after first eight weeks (before eight weeks it is called the embryo).

Fibrillation—The incoordinate contraction of muscle fibers often pertaining to the heart muscle.

Fibrinogen—Protein in blood that is converted into fibrin during blood clotting.

Free Radical—Highly reactive compound with abnormal composition of atoms and at least one unpaired electron.

Glossary

Fructose—Fruit sugar or levulose. A monosaccharide found in fruits and honey and made by hydrolysis of sucrose (table sugar).

Gastric Juice—Secretions of stomach glands containing hydrochloric acid, pepsin, mucin and, in infants, renin.

Gene—Biologic unit of heredity, part of DNA molecule.

Gingiva—Mucous membrane and connective tissue surrounding gum tissue.

Glucose—Monosaccharide found in fruits and sugars, the storage sugar of the body. The sugar found in blood, grape sugar and dextrose.

Glycogen—Animal starch, the chief storage carbohydrate in animals. Stored largely in the liver and used in the form of glucose.

Gonad—Referring to sexual organs such as female ovary or male testis.

Hemoglobin—Oxygen-carrying colored compound in the red blood cells.

Hepatic—Of or pertaining to the liver.

Histamine—Substance released from tissue during antibody reaction. May cause allergic responses.

Holistic—Referring to a philosophy that considers all aspects of human life and being integral in the assessment of an individual. Considering the physical body, emotions, mental and spiritual dimensions as being central to balanced functioning.

Homeostatis—Body's regulatory mechanism, that tries to maintain stability and consistency in various systems.

Hyperkinetic—Referring to physical overactivity.

Ileitis—Inflammation of ileum; Crohn's disease.

Ileum—Lower part of small intestine, ending before large intestine at cecum.

Infarction—Development of dead tissue resulting from obstruction of blood flow and subsequent blood flow to tissue and inability to remove waste products from area.

Intercostal—Situated between the ribs (costae).

BALANCING YOUR LIFESTYLE

Islands of Langerhans—Group of specialized cells scattered throughout the pancreas that make insulin, glucagon, etc.

Jaundice—Appearance of bile in the blood; yellow discoloration.

Keratin—Insoluble sulfur containing protein found in the skin, hair and nails.

Ketosis—Inefficient burning of fat, which alter's blood balance.

Korsakoff's Disease—Syndrome characterized by confusion, amnesia and apathy; observed in alcoholics and other B-vitamin–deficient individuals.

Kwashiorkor—Protein deficiency disease seen in malnourished children.

Lactation—The secretion of milk.

Lactose—Milk sugar; a disaccharide composed of glucose and galactose.

Legume—Seed or fruit of pod-bearing plant, including dried peas and beans, lentils, peanuts and chickpeas.

Leukocyte—A white blood cell.

Lipase—Fat emulsifying enzyme.

Lipid—Term referring to fats, including triglyceride, cholesterol and phospholipids.

Lymph—Yellowish, relatively clear fluid found in lymphatic vessels containing cells, lymphocytes, water, salts, proteins and other constituents from blood plasma.

Macronutrients—Nutrients needed by the body in large quantities, including carbohydrates, proteins, fats and water.

Maltose—A dissacharide sugar consisting of two glucose units.

Medulla—Innermost part of an organ as seen in the kidneys, adrenals and the part of the brain that connects with the spinal cord.

Melanin—Dark pigment of skin, eye and certain parts of the brain.

Meninges—The three membranes that cover the brain and spinal cord.

Glossary

Menses—Monthly flow of blood from female genital tract; menstrual cycle flow.

Metabolism—Sum total of all anabolic (building up) and catabolic (breaking down) reactions in the body.

Micronutrients—Nutrients required by the body in relatively small amounts, including vitamins and minerals.

Molecule—A minute mass of matter; the smallest particle of a chemical compound that can exist in a free state.

Monosaccharide—A simple sugar, such as glucose, fructose and galactose.

Mutagen—Substance causing genetic mutation.

Mutation—Variation in an inheritable characteristic.

Myelin—A fatlike substance that forms a covering for many nerve fibers.

Myoneural—Pertaining to motor nerve fibers.

Nephron—Structural unit of the kidney.

Neuron—Nerve cell body plus its process; structural unit of nerve tissue.

Neurotransmitter—A chemical that serves as a communication link between neurons. Usually referring to brain chemicals.

Nonessential Amino Acids—Necessary amino acids that can be synthesized by the body from amino acids in food and diet.

Norepinephrine—One of the "fight or flight" hormones related to epinephrine and derived from the amino acid tyrosine.

Nucleic Acid—Complex molecular substances, such as DNA, found in all cells to carry genetic code or responsible for protein synthesis.

Occipital—Relating to the back part of the head (the occiput).

Occlusion—Manner of closing the mouth and bringing the upper and lower teeth together; blockage in an artery, canal or vein.

Osseous—Pertaining to bone.

Ova—Female reproductive cells.

Ovulation—Discharge of mature egg cell (ovum) from the follicle of the ovary.

Oxalic acid—A dicarboxylic acid that forms insoluble salts with calcium, found in spinach, cranberries, chard and rhubarb.

Oxidation—Chemical reaction in which a substance combines with oxygen.

Pancreas—Large, elongated gland behind the stomach that aids in digestion.

Pellagra—A niacin deficiency disease characterized by skin, gastrointestinal tract and nervous system disorders.

Peristalsis—Rhythmic wavelike motion of the muscle tissue of the alimentary canal that moves the food through the digestive tube.

Phagocyte—A cell that ingests bacteria or other foreign substances.

Phenylalanine—A naturally occurring amino acid found in milk and other foods, and required for normal growth and nitrogen balance.

Phenylketonuria—Congenital deficiency of an enzyme necessary for conversion of the amino acid phenylalanine to tyrosine; characterized by mental retardation.

Photosynthesis—The process in green plants whereby chlorophyll converts the sun's energy, carbon dioxide and water into carbohydrate.

Physiology—The science that deals with the activities or functions of the body and its parts.

Pineal—Pertaining to the cone-shaped body or glandlike organ near the midbrain.

Pituitary—The "master gland," which produces hormones that regulate many body processes.

Placenta—Flat, circular organ that provides nourishment, respiration and excretion of the developing fetus.

Plaque—A deposit of fatty substances in the intima (innermost section) of the artery wall seen in atherosclerosis.

Plasma—The liquid portion of blood or lymph devoid of cells.

Glossary

Platelets—Cell fragments found in blood.

Progesterone—Female hormone that assists in female reproduction cycles and in normal development of pregnancy.

Prostaglandin—Hormonelike substances from linoleic acid and linolenic acid that affect the action of various hormones, contraction of smooth muscle and dilation of blood vessels.

Protein—A group of organic compounds consisting of carbon, hydrogen, oxygen and nitrogen (some contain sulfur and phosphorus); the principal constituent of cell protoplasm (building material of all living organisms).

Ptyalin—A starch-digesting enzyme in saliva.

Raynaud's Disease—Intermittent pallor, loss of heat from toes, fingers or both.

Renal—Pertaining to the kidney.

Retina—Innermost part of the eyeball; nerve coat of the eye.

Saponin—Emulsifying substance found in nature.

Satiety—Feeling of satisfaction after eating.

Saturated Fat—Fat or fatty acid found in animal products and some plant sources (coconut and palm oils, cocoa butter).

Semen—White, thick secretion carrying male reproductive cells (spermatozoa).

Serotonin—A neurotransmitter formed from trytophan that has a calming effect.

Serum—The fluid portion of blood that is left after clotting.

Sprue—Malabsorption syndrome characterized by poor absorption of foods and water. Symptoms are associated with nutrient deficiencies.

Steroid—Group of compounds similar to cholesterol, including bile acids, sterols and sex hormones.

Stress—The nonspecific response of the body to any demand made upon it (as defined by Hans Selye).

Subcutaneous—Below the skin.

Synovial—Relating to the thick fluid found in joints, bursae and tendon sheaths.

Systemic—Affecting the whole body.

Systole—The period of heart muscle contraction, especially that of the ventricles.

Testosterone—Male sex hormone.

Tetany—Muscle spasms due to low concentrations of calcium in the blood.

Therapy—The treatment of a disease or any disorder.

Thoracic—Relating to the chest portion of the body.

Thrombosis—Formation of a thrombus, or blood clot, that forms in the artery wall or cavity of the heart.

Thyroxine—Thyroid hormone needed for growth and proper metabolic rate.

Toxemia—General toxic condition in which poisonous bacterial products are absorbed into the bloodstream.

Trachea—Often called the "windpipe"; tube extending from the larynx to two branching bronchi of the lungs.

Triglyceride—Fatty compound composed of glycerol and fatty acids.

Trypsin—Gastric enzyme that splits protein into amino acids.

Umbilical—Relating to umbilicus or navel.

Urea—Nitrogen part of protein breakdown or metabolism excreted in the urine.

Urethra—Excretory tube of the bladder.

Uric Acid—End product of the metabolism of purines excreted in urine; generally found elevated in gout patients.

Uterus—Muscular pear-shaped organ in the female pelvis within which the fetus grows until birth.

Vaccine—A substance used to create antibodies formation.

Vagina—Lower part of female birth canal.

Varicose—Pertaining to unnatural swelling, as in the case of varix or varicose veins.

Vascular—Relating to a blood vessel.

Ventricle—One of the two lower chambers of the heart.

RESOURCES

Organic Food by Mail

Deer Valley Farm
RD #1
Guilford, NY 13780
(607) 764-8556

Ecology Sound Farms
42126 Road 168
Orosi, CA 93647
(209) 528-3816

Jordan River Farm
Huntly, VA 22640
(703) 636-9388

Mountain Ark Trading Company
120 South East Avenue
Fayetteville, AR 72701
800-643-8909

Oak Manor Farms
Tavistock, Ontario
Canada, NOB 2R0
(519) 662-2385

Pine Ridge Farms
P.O. Box 98
Subiaco, AR 72865
(501) 934-4565

Walnut Acres
Penns Creek, PA 17862
(717) 837-0601

Learning and Transformational Programs

Circle of Light Institute
505 Eighth Avenue
New York, NY 10018
(212) 564-2477

Esalen Institute
Big Sur, CA 93920
(408) 667-2335

Heartwood Healing Arts Institute
220 Harmony Lane
Garberville, CA 95440
(707) 923-2021

Himalayan Institute
RR #1 Box 400
Honesdale, PA 18431
(717) 253-5551

Kripalu Center for Yoga and Health
Box 793
Lenox, MA 01240
(413) 637-3280

Resources

New Age Center
1-3 So. Broadway
Nyack, NY 10960
(914) 353-2490

NY Open Center
83 Spring Street
New York, NY 10012
(212) 219-2527

The Omega Institute
RD #2 Box 377
Rhinebeck, NY 12572
(914) 338-6030 Sept. 15–May 15
(914) 266-4301 May 15–Sept. 15

The Wainwright House
260 Stuyvesant Avenue
Rye, NY 10680
(914) 967-6080

Helpful Hotlines

AIDS—1-800-342-AIDS
Alcohol Abuse—800-ALCOHOL
Bereavement (Compassionate Friends)—(312) 323-5010
Cancer—800-4-CANCER
Childbirth (LaMaze)—800-368-4404
Consumer Product Safety—800-638-2772
Crisis Counseling (Suicide Prevention)—(213) 381-5111
Eating Disorders—(312) 831-3438
Heart Disease—1-800-241-6993
Marriage and Family Counseling—(814) 865-1751
Second Surgical Opinion—1-800-638-6833

BALANCING YOUR LIFESTYLE

Self-Help Center—(312) 328-0470
Women's Medical Rights—(415) 826-4401
Women's Sports Foundation—800-227-3988
(212) 972-9170 (NY)

Sources of Important Health-Related Information

Alcoholics Anonymous (AA)
P.O. Box 459
Grand Central Station
New York, NY 10163

American Anorexia/Bulimia Assn.
133 Cedar Lane
Teaneck, NJ 07666
(201) 836-1800

American Cancer Society
4 West 35th Street
New York, NY 10001

American Heart Association
7320 Greenville Avenue
Dallas, TX 75231

American Holistic Medical Association
6932 Little River Turnpike
Annandale, VA 22003

ANAD (National Association of Anorexia Nervosa and
  Associated Disorders)
Box 271
Highland Park, IL 60035

Resources

Association for Applied Psychophysiology
  and Biofeedback
(Formerly: Biofeedback Society of America)
10200 West 44th St.
Wheat Ridge, CO 80033
(303) 422-8436

Center for Medical Consumers
237 Thompson Street
New York, NY 10012

Centers for Disease Control
Dept. of Health and Human Services
Atlanta, GA 30333

Commonhealth Nutrition, Inc.
P.O. Box 400
Newton Center, MA 02159

Consumers United for Food Safety
P.O. Box 22928
Seattle, WA 98122

East West Foundation
17 Station St., Box 1200
Brookline, MA 02147

Elizabeth Kübler-Ross Center
(Death, dying, bereavement)
So. Rt. 616
Headwaters, VA 2442

Exceptional Cancer Patients/Bernard Siegel, M.D.
2 Church Street South
New Haven, CT 06519
(203) 865-8392

BALANCING YOUR LIFESTYLE

The Feingold Association of the United States
Box 6550
Alexandria, VA 22306
(703) 768-FAUS

Foundation for Alternative Cancer Therapies
Box 1242, Old Chelsea Station
New York, NY 10113

Hartley Film Foundation
Cat Rock Road
Cos Cob, CT 06807

HealthComm Inc.
3215 56th St. NW
Gig Harbor, WA 98335

Health News & Review
Keats Publishing, Inc.
27 Pine Street (Box 876)
New Canaan, CT 06840

The Huxley Institution for Biosocial Research
(Newsletter, professional, journal, magazine, referral)
900 North Federal Highway
Suite 330
Boca Raton, FL 33432

Institute for Child Behavior Research
4182 Adams Avenue
San Diego, CA 92116

International Academy of Holistic Health and Medicine
Preventive Medicine Up-Date (Newsletter)
218 Avenue B
Redondo Beach, CA 90277

Resources

La Leche
9616 Minneapolis Avenue
Franklin, Park, IL 60131

Lamaze Pregnancy and Childbirth
1840 Wilson Blvd.
Arlington, VA 22201

Life-Line Nutritional Services, Inc.
c/o Joan Friedrich, Ph.D.
P.O. Box 482
Bronxville, NY 10708

National Coalition to Stop Food Irradiation
Box 59-0488
San Francisco, CA 94159

National Health Federation
P.O. Box 688
Monrovia, CA 91016

National Health Information Clearing House
U.S. Office of Disease Prevention and Health Promotion
Consumer Information Center
Pueblo, CO 81009

National Institutes of Mental Health
5600 Fishers Lane, Room 15C-05
Rockville, MD 20857

National Women's Health Network
224 7th St. S.E.
Washington, DC 20003

North American Vegetarian Society
P.O. Box 72
Dolgeville, NY 13329

Nutrition Action Health Letter
Center for Science in the Public Interest
1501 15 St. N.W.
Washington, DC 20036

Public Citizen
P.O. Box 19404
Washington, DC 20036

Walking Clubs
P.O. Box 509
Gracie Station
New York, NY 10028

Water Test Corp.
Box 186
New London, NH 03257

Whole Health Institute
4817 No. Country Rd.
Loveland, CO 80537

Rejuvenating Getaways and Escapes

Adirondack Mountain Club
174 Glen Street
Glens Falls, NY 12801

Resources

Alive Polarity at Murietta Hot Springs
28779 Via Las Flores
Murietta, CA 92362
(714) 677-7451

American Youth Hostels
75 Spring Street
New York, NY 10012
(212) 421-7100

Bermuda Inn
43019 Sierra Highway
Lancaster, CA 93534
(805) 942-1492
Toll Free in California: 1-800-328-3276

Beverly Antaeus
Women's Canoe Trips
P.O. Box 9109
Santa Fe, NM 87504
(505) 984-2268

Bonaventure Resort and Spa
250 Racquet Club Rd.
Ft. Lauderdale, FL 33326

Boojum Expeditions
Box 2236
Leucadia, CA 92024
(619) 435-3927

Butterfield & Robinson
70 Bond Street
Toronto, Canada M5B 1X3

BALANCING YOUR LIFESTYLE

Canyon Ranch Health and Fitness Resort
Tucson, AZ

Country Cycling Tours
140 West 83rd Street
New York, NY 10024
(212) 874-5151

Crystal Journeys
Joseph Cohen
P.O. Box 7228A
Toronto, Ontario, Canada
M5W 1XS
(416) 967-6195
(416) 626-5465

Desert Palms Wellness Institute
120 W. Hilton Drive
St. George, UT 84770
(801) 628-4140

Diet Holiday Resort
Regent House
2000 So. Ocean Drive/Dept. C.
Hallandale, FL 33039

Earthstar
174 Whitehall Rd. R 12
Hooksett, NH 03106
(603) 669-9497

Earthwatch
680 Mount Auburn Street
Box 403
Watertown, MA 02172
(617) 926-8200

Resources

Hilton Head Health Institute
P.O. Box 7138
Hilton Head Island, SC 29938
(803) 785-7292

Journeys
1120 Clair Circle
Ann Arbor, MI 48103
(313) 665-4407

Lake Austin Resort
1705 Quinlan Park Rd.
Austin, TX 78732
(512) 266-2444
800-252-9324

Mohonk Mountain House
Mohonk Lake
New Paltz, NY 12561
(914) 255-1000
(212) 233-2244

Mountain Workshops
P.O. Box 625
Ridgefield, CT 06877

Murrieta Hot Springs Vegetarian Oasis
28779 Via Las Flores P-8
Murrieta, CA 92362
(714) 677-7451

New Age Health Farm
Neversink, NY 12765
(914) 985-2221

BALANCING YOUR LIFESTYLE

New Life Spa
Liftline Lodge
Stratton Mt., VT 05155
(802) 297-2534

Northern Pines Health Resort
Route 85, Box 279
Raymond, ME 04071
(207) 655-7624

Norwich Inn and Spa
Rte. 32
Norwich, CT 06360

Odyssey Tours
1821 Wilshire Blvd.
Santa Monica, CA 90403
(213) 453-1042
1-800-654-7975

Palm Aire Hotel and Spa
2501 Palm-Aire Drive
Pompano Beach, FL 33069
800-327-4960

The Palms
572 North Indian Avenue
Palm Springs, CA 92262
(619) 325-1111

Pawling Health Manor
Box 401
Hyde Park, NY 12539
(914) 889-4141

Resources

Pocono Whitewater Rafting Center
Route 903
Jim Thorpe, PA 18229
(717) 325-3656

Progressive Travels, Ltd.
P.O. Box 775164
Steamboat Springs, CO 80477
(303) 879-2859 (Colorado)
1-800-245-2229 (nationwide)

Rancho Rio Caliente
Guadalajara, Jalisco, Mexico
For information contact:
Barbara Dane Associates
480 California Terrace
Pasadena, CA 91105
(818) 796-5577

Rocky Mountain Wellness Spa
Box 777
Steamboat Springs, CO 80477
(303) 879-7772

Russell House of Key West
611 Truman Avenue
Key West, FL 33040
(305) 294-8787

Safety Harbor Spa Fitness Center
105 No. Bayshore Drive
Safety Harbor, FL 33572
800-237-0155

BALANCING YOUR LIFESTYLE

Shangri-La Natural Health Resort
Bonita Springs, FL 33923
(813) 992-3811

Sharon Springs Health Spa
Chestnut Street
Sharon Springs, NY 13459
(518) 284-2885

Sierra Club
217 E. 85th Street, Suite 200
New York, NY 10028

Spa at Waterville Valley
Box CS
Waterville Valley, NH 03223
1-800-258-8988
1-800-552-4767 (in NH)

Su Casa
Rte 28A
West Hurley, NY 12491

Tiberti Travel, Ltd.
177 East 87th Street, Ste. 401
New York, NY 10128
(212) 427-5913
1-800-227-6772

Turnwood Organic Gardens
HCRI Box 62
Lew Beach, NY 12753
(914) 439-5702

Resources

Turnwood Gardens Retreat
Turnwood Star Route
Livingston Manor, NY 12758

Vegetarian Hotel
P.O. Box 457
Woodridge, NY 12789
(914) 434-4455

Vermont Bicycle Touring
Box 711
Briston, VT 05443
(802) 453-4811

White Cloud
RD 1 Box 215
Newfoundland, PA 18445
(717) 676-3162

Windjammer Barefoot Cruises
P.O. Box 120
Miami Beach, FL 33119-9990
(305) 373-2090
1-800-327-2601 (outside Florida)
1-800-432-3364 (inside Florida)

REFERENCES

American Heart Association, Cooking Without Your Salt Shaker.

American Holistic Medical Associations, Nutritional Guidelines, Kozora, E.J. (editor) AHMA, Annandale, Va.

Asterita, M. (1985), *The Physiology of Stress*. New York: Human Sciences, Press.

Bedford, S. (1980), *Stress and Tiger Juice*. Chico, Calif.: Scott Publications.

Bland, J. (ed.) (1985, 1986), *1984–1985, and 1986 Yearbook of Nutritional Medicine*. New Canaan, Conn.: Keats Publishing.

Braverman, E. & Pfeiffer, C.C. (1986), *The Healing Nutrients Within: Facts, Findings and New Research on Amino Acids*. New Canaan, Conn.: Keats Publishing.

Brody, J. (1981), *Jane Brody's Nutrition Book*. New York: W.W. Norton.

Clark, C.C. (1981), *Enhancing Wellness: A Guide for Self-Care*. New York: Springer Publishing Co.

Copper, K.H. (1982), *The Aerobics Program for Total Well-Being*. New York: M. Evans.

Feingold, B. (1986), *The Feingold Handbook*. Alexandria, Va. (1985), Feingold Association of the United States.

Garrison, R. & Somer, E. (1985), *The Nutrition Desk Reference*. New Canaan, Conn.: Keats Publishing.

References

Holmes, T.H., & Rahe, R.H. (1967), The Social Readjustment Rating Scale. *Journal of Psychosomatic Research*, New York: 1:213–218.

Krilanovila, N. *No Sugar Added, or Redesigning Our Children's Future*. Santa Barbara, Calif.: November Books.

Kugler, H. (1985), *The Anti-Aging Weight Loss Program*. New York: Stein and Day.

McCaull, J. & Crossland, J. (1974), *Water Pollution*. New York: Harcourt Brace Jovanovich, Inc.

Memmler, R.L. & Wood, D.L. (1977), *Structure and Function of the Human Body*, 2d ed. Philadelphia, Pa.: J.B. Lippincott.

Nuernberger, P. (1983), *Freedom from Stress*. Honesdale, Pa.: Himalayan International Institute.

Nutrition Action Health Letter. Center for Science in the Public Interest. Volume 12, No. 9, Volume 14, No. 1, Volume 13, No. 11.

Patient Medication Bulletin (1986), P.O. Box 14281, Torrance, Calif. 90503.

Pelletier, K. (1977), *Mind as Healer, Mind as Slayer*. New York: Dell Publishing.

Pennington, J. & Church, H.N. (1985), *Food Values of Portions Commonly Used*. 14th ed. New York: Harper and Row.

Public Citizen Health Research Group (1984), #992, Food Additive Report, Washington, D.C.

Public Citizen Health Research Group (1986), Food Irradiation: The Other Side of the Story, Washington, D.C.

Quigley, D.T. (1981), *National Malnutrition*. Baton Rouge, La.: B of A Communications.

Robinson, C.H. (1982), *Normal and Therapeutic Nutrition*, 14th ed. New York: Macmillan.

Schiff Nutrition Alert, Vol. 2, #2, FDA (DHS), Nov. 20, 1985, Consumer Letter.

Schroeder, M.D. (1974), *The Poisons Around Us*. New Canaan, Conn.: Keats Publishing.

Selye, H. (1977). *Stress Without Distress.* Philadelphia, Pa.: J.B. Lippincott.

Stewart, M.A. (1970), Hyperactive Children. *Scientific American*, 222:94–98.

────── et al. (1966), The Hyperactive Child Syndrome. *Am. Journal of Orthomolecular Psychiatry*, 36:861–867.

USDA Human Nutrition Information Service (1986), Nutrition and Your Health: Dietary Guidelines for Americans.

US Dept. of Health & Human Services. The 1984 Report of the Joint National Committee on the Detection, Evaluations and Treatment of High Blood Pressure: National Institutes of Health Publication. #84-1088. Sept. 1984. (Also published in *Archives of Internal Medicine*, Vol. 144, May 1984.)

US Dept. of Health and Human Services, National Institute on Alcohol Abuse and Alcoholism, Rockville, Md.

INDEX

ACTH, 76
Additives, 7–8, 21–22
  avoidance of, 22
  common sodium food additives, 19–20
Aerobic exercise, 64, 66–67
Alcohol, 30–33
  consumption during pregnancy, 31
  contents in common beverages, 31
  legal intoxication, 32–33
Allergies, 34–42
  common symptoms of, 36–37
  to food families, 37–39
  understanding, 35–36
  to yeast, 39–40
American Heart Association, 16
Amino acids, 54–57
  common food sources of, 56–57
  essential and nonessential, 55
Anaerobic exercise, 67
Antigens, 36
Anxiety, drugs for, 74
Artificial colors, 21, 22
Artificial sweeteners, 21, 22
Asthma, 41–42

Balance, concept of, 3
Basal metabolic rate, raising, 66
Beans, 46
  cooking methods for, 25

Beverages
  alcohol content of, 31
  caffeine content of, 29
  healthful, 47
BHA/BHT, 21, 22
Biofeedback, 83
Blood alcohol content, 32–33
Blood cholesterol. *See* Cholesterol
Blood pressure, normal ranges of, 18
Body measurements, 70
Brain damage, alcohol and, 31
Breads, 46
Breathing, directions for complete, 83–85
Breathing phrases, 85

Caffeine, 27–29
  in common beverages, 29
  effects of, 28
  in nonprescription drugs, 29
Calories
  activities that burn, 68–69
  for weight loss and optimum health, 72
Cancer
  additives and, 21, 22
  alcohol and, 31
  carcinogenic by-products of treated food, 26
  carcinogens in water, 30
  cholesterol and, 17
  weight and, 71

Candida albicans, 40
Candidiasis, 40
Carbohydrates, healthful, 48
Carcinogens. *See* Cancer
Cardiomyopathy, 31
Cardiovascular disease. *See also* Heart disease
    blood pressure and, 18
Cereals, 46
Chemical preservatives, 21–22
Children
    blood cholesterol guidelines for, 17
    characteristics of well-nourished, 10
Cholesterol
    blood cholesterol guidelines for children and adults, 17
    cancer and, 17
    in common foods, 16–17
    fiber and, 50
    heart disease and, 16
Cirrhosis of the liver, 30
Coffee, 27–28
Condiments, healthful, 47
Cooking, suggested methods of, 25
Counseling, stress management and, 80–81

Deficiency disease, 50
Degenerative diseases, 8
Diabetes, weight and, 71
Diet
    disease and, 2
    risks of a declining, 7–8
    Senate Select Committee recommendations for, 9
    structuring, 48–49
    for weight control and optimum health, 72
Disease(s)
    deficiency, 50
    degenerative, 8
    personality type and, 82
    stress and, 73
    weight and, 71
Distilled water, 30
Distress, 76
Drinking water, 30

Drugs
    monoamine oxidase inhibitor (MAO) drugs, 59–60
    nonprescription, 29
    role in destroying supplements, 57–58
    sulfite-containing, 41

Emergency breathing, 83
Emotions, health and, 78
Essential amino acids, 54
Ethylene dibromide (EDB), 26
Eustress, 76
Exercise
    aerobic, 64, 66–67
    anaerobic, 67
    for breathing, 83–85
    forms of, 66–68
    pulse rate during, 66
    weight control and, 68–69

Fast foods, 15
Fats, 13–17, 49
    in the American diet, 13
    percentages in common foods, 14–16
Feingold, Benjamin, 34
Fetus, alcohol and, 31
Fiber, 50
Fish, 47
Flour products, processed, 43
Food
    allergies to, 37–39
    containing yeast, 40
    foods to avoid, 43–44
    healthful, 44–48
    insecticide-treated or irradiated, 25–27
    nutrients lost in refining, 24
    overprocessed and overcooked, 24–25
    suggested cooking methods, 25
    treatment of, 7–8
Food additives. *See* Additives
Food and Drug Administration (FDA), 41, 42
Food dyes, 22
Food supplements. *See also* Minerals; Vitamins
    drugs and, 57–58

Fruits, 45
Fumigants, 26

Gastritis, alcohol and, 31
Generally recognized as safe (GRAS), 41
Grains, 46
  cooking methods for, 25

Happiness, mental health and, 78
Headache, dietary restrictions for, 59–60
Health. See also Wellness
  weight and, 71
Heart attack, personality type and, 82
Heart disease, 8
  alcohol and, 30–31
  weight and, 71
Heart rate, 64–66
High-density lipoproteins (HDL), 14
Histamines, 36
Holistic medicine, 2
Hormones, stress and, 77
Hydrogenated oils, 13
Hyperactive children, 28

Immune system, allergies and, 35–36
Ingredients, labeling of, 11–12
Insecticide-treated food, 25–26
Intoxication, 32–33
Irradiated food, 25–27
Isokinetic exercise, 67–68
Isometric exercise, 67
Isophasic exercise, 67
Isotonic exercise, 67

Junk food, 15

Labeling of ingredients, 11–12
Legumes, cooking methods for, 25
Life events, stress and, 74–75
Liver, effects of alcohol on, 30
Low-density lipoproteins (LDL), 14

Malnutrition, 8
  alcohol and, 31
MAO. See Monoamine oxidase.

Meat, 47
  fat content of, 14–16
Men, weight recommendations for, 69
Mental illness, warning signs of, 77
Menu, sample healthful, 49
Metals, toxic, 22–24
Migraine patients, dietary restrictions for, 59–60
Minerals, 50–51, 53–54
Monoamine oxidase (MAO) inhibitor drugs, 59–60
Monounsaturated oils, 13–14

Neustress, 76
Nonprescription drugs, caffeine in, 29
Nuts, 46–47

Obesity, 8
Oils, 13–14, 46–47

Perception, role in controlling stress, 80
Personality type, stress and, 82
Pollution, of water, 29–30
Polyunsaturated oils, 13
Poultry, 47
Pregnancy, alcohol consumption during, 31
Preservatives, 21–22
Processed foods, 21–22, 24–25
  salt content in, 18
Proteins, 48
  amino acids and, 54–56
  vegetarian, 44
Psychosomatic illness, 78
Psychotherapy, stress management and, 80–81
Pulse rate, during exercise, 66

Relaxation
  breathing and, 85
  stress and, 83
Resting heart rate, 65–66

Saccharin, 22
Salicylates, 34
  naturally occurring, 35

Salt, 18–21
  danger of excess, 18
  salt-sodium conversions, 19
  seasoning food without, 20–21
Saturated fats, 13
Seasonings, 20–21
Sea vegetables, 46
Sedatives, 74
Seeds, 46–47
Shopping list, healthful, 45–48
Snacks, healthful, 47–48
Social readjustment scale, 74–75
Sodium, 18–21
  common high-sodium foods, 19
  common sodium food additives, 19–20
Sodium nitrate, 22
Stress, 44
  breathing and, 83–85
  health and, 73–74
  life stressors, 74–77
  social readjustment scale, 74–75
  ways to diminish, 82–83
Stress indicators, 79
Stress management, 80–81
Stroke, weight and, 71
Sugar, 11–13, 43
  alternative names for, 11
  foods high in, 12
Sulfites, 41–42
  adverse reactions to, 41
  foods containing, 42

Supplements. *See also* Minerals; Vitamins
  drugs and, 57–58
Symptoms, importance of, 2

Tap water, 29–30
Toxic metals, 22–24, 22–24
Trace metals, toxic, 23–24
Training heart rate, 64–65
Type A personality, characteristics of, 81
Type B personality, characteristics of, 81
Tyramine, 59–60

Ulcers, alcohol and, 31

Vegetables
  cooking methods for, 25
  types of, 45
Vegetarian proteins, 44
Vitamins, 50–53

Water, pollution of, 29–30
Weight
  control of through exercise, 68–69
  health and, 71
Weight loss, indications for, 70
Weight recommendations, 69
Wellness, understanding, 1–3
Women, weight recommendations for, 69

Yeast
  allergies and, 39–40
  yeast-containing foods, 40